The Thyroid Sourcebook

The Thyroid Sourcebook

5th Edition

M. Sara Rosenthal, Ph.D.

New York   Chicago   San Francisco   Lisbon   London   Madrid   Mexico City
Milan   New Delhi   San Juan   Seoul   Singapore   Sydney   Toronto

Library of Congress Cataloging-in-Publication Data

Rosenthal, M. Sara.
    The thyroid sourcebook / M. Sara Rosenthal.—5th ed.
        p.   cm.
    Includes bibliographical references.
    ISBN-13: 978-0-07-159725-8 (alk. paper)
    ISBN-10: 0-07-159725-5 (alk. paper)
    1. Thyroid gland—Popular works.   I. Title.

   RC655.R67   2009
   616.4'4—dc22   2008034450

3 4 5 6 7 8 9 10 11 12 13 14 15 16 17 18 19   FGR/FGR   0

ISBN 978-0-07-159725-8
MHID   0-07-159725-5

McGraw-Hill books are available at special quantity discounts to use as premiums and sales promotions or for use in corporate training programs. To contact a representative, please visit the Contact Us pages at www.mhprofessional.com.

The information in this book is intended to provide helpful and informative material on the subject addressed. It is not intended to serve as a replacement for professional medical advice. Any use of the information in this book is at the reader's discretion. The author and publisher specifically disclaim any and all liability arising directly or indirectly from the use or application of any information contained in this book. A health-care professional should be consulted regarding your specific situation.

This book is printed on acid-free paper.

To my maternal grandparents
Jacob Lander, M.D. (1910–1989)
Clara Lander, Ph.D. (1916–1978)

Contents

Acknowledgments   xi
Introduction: Arming Yourself with
  Thyroid Health Information   xiii

1 Meet Your Thyroid Gland: A Beautiful Butterfly   1

How Your Thyroid Works   2
Thyroid Disorders and Treatments: An Overview   9

2 Slowing Down: Hypothyroidism   13

Symptoms of Hypothyroidism   14
Diagnosing Hypothyroidism   19
Common Causes of Hypothyroidism   21
Treating Hypothyroidism   27
Feeling Hypothyroid When Your Tests Are Normal   27

3 Speeding Up: Thyrotoxicosis and Hyperthyroidism   33

Signs of Thyrotoxicosis   33
Graves' Disease: The Most Common Cause of
  Hyperthyroidism   43

Other Causes of Thyrotoxicosis   51
Diagnosing Thyrotoxicosis and/or Hyperthyroidism   53
Treating Thyrotoxicosis Not Caused by Graves' Disease   54

4   **Thyroiditis: Inflammation of the Thyroid Gland**   57

Subacute Viral Thyroiditis: Pain in the Neck!   57
Silent Thyroiditis   59
Postpartum Thyroiditis   60
Acute Suppurative Thyroiditis   61
Riedel's Thyroiditis   62

5   **Thyroid Nodules: Lumps in the Thyroid Gland**   63

Finding a Thyroid Nodule   64
Evaluating a Nodule   66
Types of Thyroid Nodules   70
Who Should Be Screened for Thyroid Nodules?   77

6   **Thyroid Cancer: A Beginner's Guide**   81

What Causes Thyroid Cancer?   81
Signs of Thyroid Cancer   83
Types of Thyroid Cancer   85
Staging and Spreading   87
Treating Common Types of Thyroid Cancer   89
What You Should Know About Thyroidectomy   90
Follow-Up Scans and Tests   94
Thyroid Hormone Suppression Therapy   95
Treating Recurrence   96

7   **Complications, Other Conditions, and Comorbidities:
    When Other Stuff Happens, Too**   97

Thyroid Eye Disease   97
Depression or Anxiety: Could It Be My Thyroid?   102
Heart Disease and Thyroid Disease: A
  Troublesome Duo   106
Fatigue: Sleep Disorder or Thyroid Disease?   112

Menopause and Thyroid Disease   116
Thyroid Disease After Sixty   118
The Autoimmune Disease Collection Package   120

8   Thyroid Disease and New Life: Fertility, Pregnancy,
    Postpartum, and Neonatal Issues   121

    Thyroid Disease and Fertility   122
    Normal Pregnancy Discomforts: How They Relate
      to Thyroid Disease   124
    Pregnancy and Preexisting Thyroid Disease   125
    Gestational Thyroid Disease   126
    Discovering Thyroid Nodules During Pregnancy   130
    After the Baby Is Born   130
    Thyroid Disease in Newborns and Infants   133

9   Hot Stuff: A Beginner's Guide to Radioactive Iodine   137

    What Is Radioactive Iodine?   138
    Nuclear Testing with Radioactive Iodine   139
    Radioactive Iodine Treatment   143

10 Helping the Medicine Go Down: Thyroid Hormone
    Replacement and Other Medications   153

    A Brief History of Thyroid Hormone Replacement   154
    Synthetic Versus "Natural" Thyroid Hormone:
      A Reality Check   154
    Twenty-First-Century Thyroid Hormone Therapy   157
    When You Must Take T3   164

11 What to Eat: Diet, Nutrition, and Thyroid Disease 169

    Diet and Iodine   169
    The Low-Iodine Diet   173
    The Hypothyroid Diet for Life: Low Glycemic Index,
      Low Fat, and High Fiber   178
    The Hyperthyroid Diet   183
    Thyroid Disease and Obesity   183

12   Complementary Activities and Therapies: When You Need a Massage — **187**

Becoming Active — 187
For Your Mental Health — 191
Feel-Good Therapies That Work! — 197

Appendix A: How to Assess Thyroid Books, Websites, and Other Resources — 203
Appendix B: Legitimate Thyroid Resources for Patients — 211
Glossary — 217
Bibliography — 229
Index — 235

Acknowledgments

I'D LIKE TO thank the late Robert Volpé, M.D., F.R.C.P., F.A.C.P., who served as medical adviser on the first edition of this book; my colleagues at the American Thyroid Association and The Endocrine Society; and my husband, Kenneth B. Ain, M.D., Professor of Medicine and Director, Thyroid Oncology Program, Division of Endocrinology & Molecular Medicine, Department of Internal Medicine, University of Kentucky Medical Center, who served as medical adviser of this new edition.

Sarah Pelz, my editor at McGraw-Hill, believed it was time to revise this book for a new generation of thyroid patients, and my publisher, Judith McCarthy, continues to champion my efforts in thyroid health books.

Introduction

Arming Yourself with Thyroid Health Information

WELCOME TO THE fifth edition of *The Thyroid Sourcebook*, which continues to be the classic primer on thyroid disease for thyroid patients. This new edition is completely revised for a new era in thyroid health information.

How *The Thyroid Sourcebook* Came to Be

Writing *The Thyroid Sourcebook* was inspired in large part by my own experiences. In 1983, as a twenty-year-old undergraduate student, I saw a poster put out by the Canadian Cancer Society while sitting on the Toronto subway. The poster alerted the readers to signs of cancer, one of which was a lump on the neck. I had a golf-ball-size lump just under my ear. My family doctor chose to ignore it and said many people have lumps: "Let's wait and see if it gets smaller." I went back a month later and was sent to a plastic surgeon. The plastic surgeon told me he would remove it under a local anesthetic, an excisional biopsy.

Had I known then what I know now, I would have done things much differently. I would have expected more and been better informed. When the procedure was performed, for example, I was not given an appropriate amount of local anesthetic—I could feel the procedure. I was also not given any pain medication following the procedure, and I felt a lot of pain as a result.

Finally, when the lump was found to be cancerous, the doctor told my mother instead of me. Even in 1983, this was an outrageous way to manage a thyroid cancer diagnosis for a twenty-year-old woman, breaching common ethical principles such as informed consent and confidentiality. My mother started her sentence with, "They found a malignancy." I listened to her sputter on awkwardly before I realized she was talking about *me* and not herself.

I went through the treatment process with almost no information. I had a total thyroidectomy, neck dissection, postsurgery numbness, and the appropriate scans, after first being made hypothyroid. After my first radioactive iodine therapy, I was told I would need external beam radiation therapy. This was the most exhausting and painful part of the treatment. I had daily treatments for a month, but I was not prepared for the side effects of a very sore throat and a severe sunburn on the squared-off area of my neck. I still have a color difference as a result.

What continues to haunt me is how ignorant I was throughout the whole process. Only twenty years later did I learn that I likely had an aggressive tall cell papillary cancer that had lost the ability to suck up iodine. This is why they referred me for external beam therapy. All my scans since have been clean; my thyroglobulin remains undetectable. I had a very good surgeon and good initial treatment. My follow-up, as I have learned more recently, was not optimal, but I believe the external beam therapy saved my life.

Nineteen eighty-three was the pre-Internet age and even pre-PC (unless you count the Commodore 64). People who needed information bought books or went to the library. At that time, there were no nontechnical thyroid books for patients. There were a handful of physician-authored books, but most patients found them to be too brief in some areas and too technical in others. Information about thyroid cancer was completely absent from all the patient literature at that time. Thyroid foundations for patients had just emerged, but none of my doctors pointed me to such foundations.

After I was treated for my thyroid cancer, I graduated from university with a degree in English Literature and became a journalist with health as my focus. In the early 1990s I wrote and researched a magazine article on thyroid disease and decided then that a book for thyroid patients—from the patient's perspective—ought to be written, considering that there was a paltry quantity of patient literature available on thyroid disease. I wanted to write the book I wished I had when I was first diagnosed. This idea eventually blossomed into *The Thyroid Sourcebook*, first published in 1993.

The original edition of *The Thyroid Sourcebook* benefited from the medical advisor for the project, Dr. Robert Volpé. A great thyroid expert who has since passed away, Dr. Volpé is best known for his research in the areas of autoimmune thyroid disease. With his guidance, I was free to create a work that explained things in plain language for patients who, like me, did not have the medical and science backgrounds necessary to understand "Medical Speak" and make informed decisions. The book caught on quickly with patients and was soon recommended by Jane E. Brody, a health columnist at the *New York Times*, as well as by doctors.

As the first guide for thyroid patients, the book established itself as a trusted source for accurate, easy-to-understand information. For a long time, *The Thyroid Sourcebook* was the only detailed, nontechnical book readily available in bookstores to thyroid patients. Over the years, this book had been revised four times and became one of the most stolen library books!

In the mid-1990s, as my health journalism career flourished and I wrote many more health books, I became interested in a new field that was just emerging: bioethics. I completed my master's and doctorate in bioethics, joined the faculty at The University of Kentucky as a bioethicist, and began to publish in the peer-reviewed (academic) literature on thyroid ethics—a territory no bioethicist had ventured into before.

The Challenges of Being a Thyroid Patient Today

Despite the advances in medicine, awareness, and technology since *The Thyroid Sourcebook* was first published, it's just as difficult—if not more so—to find accurate information as a thyroid patient today than it ever was. Thyroid disease went from an orphan topic in the 1990s to a saturated health market by 2001. In the late 1990s, as the Internet became much more accessible and popular, thyroid patients began surfing for thyroid information; thyroid websites and listserves abounded. But, as numerous studies have shown, the information available on the majority of health websites is dubious and highly variable.

The illusion of expertise that is created from simply "being in print" is powerful. Anyone can publish unedited health content. This excess of misinformation is problematic for thyroid patients with no medical background who are suffering from the symptoms of thyroid disease; in fact, it can create just as many problems for patients as no information at all. So while the Internet indeed helped to correct the absence of information, it created a different problem: too much inaccurate information. Today, thyroid patients emerge from an Internet search with more incorrect information than correct information. Although there are plenty of credible sources of thyroid information online, they are lost in a sea of other websites with questionable content. This is affecting thyroid patient care globally.

Thyroid Chatrooms, Listserves, and Blogs

Website chatrooms are a magnet for the thyroid patient who has not been able to get appropriate care or enough information to make informed decisions. Thousands of thyroid patients with good and bad experiences are telling their stories online. This can be validating for other patients, but a lot of this material misinterprets all kinds of medical facts—creating false facts that sound true. It's not unusual to read about bad experiences thirdhand, as in, "My sister's girlfriend had hypothyroidism and her doctor said . . ."

The Alternative Thyroid E-Health Movement

The growth of the alternative health movement coincided with the growth of the Internet, as well as with the problematic 1994 legislation allowing deregulation of dietary supplements, herbal products, and other nutraceuticals in the United States. This led to a "virtual" explosion of alternative health selling and pedaling to vulnerable patients in all health sectors. Some popular thyroid websites began to shift focus to the alternative medicine approach to thyroid disease—alternative meaning anything that was not mainstream or conventional standard of care. As a result, many websites began to promote discredited theories and treatments, publishing the opinions of questionably trained providers who claimed to specialize in thyroid disease but in reality were either not recognized by their clinical peers as appropriately trained experts or not recognized as published experts in the peer-reviewed literature.

What began to occur was widespread endorsement of unconventional natural therapies and outdated diagnostic procedures as safer and better than the standard of care. A significant portion of thyroid patient literature encourages patients to stay away from conventional endocrinologists and look for alternative health practitioners to obtain the best thyroid health care.

People selling alternative health services and products often zero in on thyroid patients as the perfect market because their health problems are so diffuse: fatigue, weight gain, anxiety, depression, metabolic problems, and so forth. Alternative health retailers are frequently disguised as "experts."

A common practice is "trick to click." Here, newsletters may be sent to your inbox with sensationalized headlines with a "Read more" URL link. The more hits a website gets, the higher its Google placement. Google searches may also send you through a thread of links that are all connected to the same websites. In some cases, "trick to click" generates revenue, as some website page authors are paid by the hit.

In other examples, tempting information packets, newsletter subscriptions, and other suspect content may be sold when the website's free content convinces you that these documents are the answer to your ailments. Some websites sell expensive consultations; in one case, a thyroid patient with no medical training charged patients for her health advice as a "patient advocate," which, according to several state laws, amounts to practicing medicine without a license. Some thyroid retailers sell self-testing kits and specially compounded "thyroid hormone" formulations (we'll get to this in Chapter 10). This translates into millions of dollars for the retailers, while thyroid patients are cruelly manipulated. Ironically, thyroid patients are often told by these same retailers that their doctors are all "in the pockets" of pharmaceutical companies and so should not be trusted, while lining their own pockets with patients' money.

A Crisis in Thyroid Patient Care

What is clear is this: The incidence of thyroid disease is dramatically rising, prompting patients to seek out information on thyroid disease. The more information thyroid patients access, the less accurate information they frequently have. Thyroid sufferers remain confused. Armed with more false information than real medical facts, many thyroid patients are at risk. And their relationships with their doctors are often at risk as well, because doctors can become frustrated spending time educating patients regarding the false information they have been reading online.

Thyroid health misinformation always existed; when I wrote the first edition of this book in 1991–1992, the fake thyroid disease Wilson's thyroid syndrome (see Chapter 2) was all the rage, for example. But the Internet has turned misinformation into what I call a new kind of thyroid virus that has spread—virtually—everywhere. The popularity of thyroid health on the Internet has also fed the thyroid misinformation book market; there are now dozens of popular thyroid books that contain content that directs thyroid patients to questionable tests and treatments. This is leading to a crisis in patient care that creates "misinformed consent" for patients and frustrated doctors. All the while, the patient population is rising faster than the pool of thyroid experts being trained to look after them.

A Shrinking Pool of Thyroid Doctors

As of this writing, there are not enough thyroid experts in North America to handle the increase in thyroid disease. First, the pool of endocrinologists all over North America is shrinking. Senior and experienced thyroid experts in the United States are struggling to find younger doctors to train and eventually hand over their practices to. In my own university, the director of our Endocrine Fellows program (a fellow is a doctor who has finished residency who then completes one to two years of extra training in his or her specialty) confided to me that he struggles to find qualified fellows who have trained in the United States. Many of our doctors are now foreign-trained, because education is subsidized in most other parts of the world.

Out of that shrinking pool of endocrinologists, most will choose diabetes, not thyroid disease, as their area of focus. When doctors see ten diabetes patients for every one thyroid patient, the level of expertise in thyroid disease may vary greatly—especially for patients with more complex needs. This makes it even harder for patients to get the medical care they need.

My Goals for You

Without enough doctors to serve the patient population and with misinformation abounding, thyroid patients deserve to understand and appreciate the differences between proven, standard-of-care therapies and unproven, experimental therapies that can be dangerous. Right now, most patients are navigating in the dark.

As a bioethicist, thyroid health author, and longtime thyroid patient, I find what's emerging in thyroid patient care very concerning. As the first patient voice for thyroid patients (going strong for more than fifteen years), it's time to speak up again.

This completely revised edition of the original trusted source for thyroid disease will give you accurate, evidence-based information—including evidence-based *complementary* therapies; provide unique information you won't find elsewhere; and address misinformation you may have read on the Internet or in other books. Woven through are stories collected from other thyroid patients (names and identifiers have been changed) to give you real case studies. To complement your Internet searches, I've added an appendix with surfing lessons (see Appendix A) so you can navigate the Internet safely for accurate information. To correct common myths and false facts, I've added a "Be Informed" sidebar with an icon 🦋 that sheds light on misinformation and helps you to be a better-informed patient.

Ultimately, my goal is the same now as it was when I first wrote this book in 1993: to set you on the right path for understanding thyroid disease so that you can make informed decisions and live better, happier, and healthier lives with thyroid disease.

The Thyroid Sourcebook

1

Meet Your Thyroid Gland

A Beautiful Butterfly

AN ENDOCRINOLOGIST IN South Dakota shared a story that illustrates how in the dark most of us are about our thyroid glands. He was treating a new patient for a thyroid condition and explained what the thyroid gland is, how it works, and what it does. The patient was fascinated by this new, critical body part she never realized she had and asked the doctor, "Do cows have thyroid glands? Or other animals?" "Yes," he answered, "all animals, fish, birds, and most other species have thyroid glands." As a newly practicing endocrinologist, he was surprised that this patient was completely unaware of her thyroid gland. But this is not unusual—most people are not aware of their thyroid glands unless they are diagnosed with a thyroid disorder.

Approximately 12 percent of the entire adult population worldwide suffers from some sort of thyroid disease. In the United States, this translates into roughly thirty million adults. Thyroid diseases are grouped by type, such as hypothyroidism, hyperthyroidism, and thyroid cancer. Twenty percent of all women will develop autoimmune thyroid disease, usually hypothyroidism, at some time in their life. Nearly one-fifth of all people over sixty have subclinical hypothyroidism, or mild hypothyroidism.

The purpose of this chapter is to describe where the thyroid gland is located, what it does, and how it works. It also briefly explains the most common thyroid disorders. In addition, it addresses some com-

1

mon misinformation that can interfere with proper decision making regarding your thyroid health. (For information on how to evaluate whether the information you find in various sources is correct, see Appendix A.) The idea is to provide you with enough information about the thyroid gland so you can better understand your diagnosis and make fully informed treatment decisions with your doctor. Since this chapter serves as a very general introduction to the thyroid gland, it will refer you to other chapters in the book for more details.

How Your Thyroid Works

The thyroid gland is often referred to as a butterfly-shaped gland, but it is also shaped like the capital letter H, specifically, the H of the Honda vehicle logo. Each side of the H or butterfly is called a lobe, while the center (the body of the butterfly) is called the isthmus. The thyroid gland is located in the lower part of your neck, in front of your windpipe, and is basically wrapped around the windpipe (see Figure 1.1). Using the butterfly analogy, the butterfly "hugs" the windpipe.

Figure 1.1

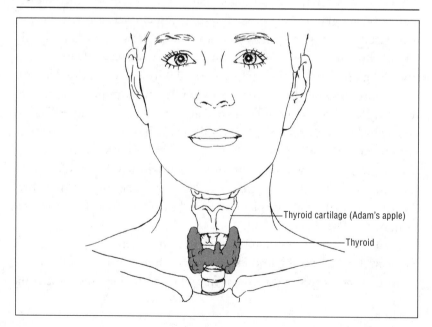

Thyroid cartilage (Adam's apple)

Thyroid

The thyroid gland makes two critical thyroid hormones. The first is thyroxine, known as T4, which has four iodine atoms for each hormone molecule. The second is triiodothyronine, or T3, which has three iodine atoms for each hormone molecule. Both hormones are referred to in the singular as thyroid hormone.

Thyroid hormone is essential for our existence, affecting every single cell in the body. Thyroid hormone serves as the speed control for our cells, controlling their "speed of life." Of the two hormones, it is thought that only T3 has a direct effect on the cells of the body; it is debatable whether T4 has any direct effect. T4 must be converted to T3 by the cells by removing one specific iodine atom before it can work. If a different iodine atom is removed from T4, it creates an inactive molecule that does not work as an effective thyroid hormone. Nearly all cells have special enzymes inside of them called deiodinases that remove the iodine atom from T4 to make it into T3. It is thought that this is one way that each cell customizes how much T3 it will get, even though the blood supply to all the cells generally provides the same level of T4 at the same time. The T3 produced in the body's cells works in the nucleus of these cells to turn some genes on and some genes off. This is how the thyroid hormone works in the body.

For example, in the cells of the pituitary gland (where thyroid-stimulating hormone (TSH) is produced), T3 turns off the gene that makes TSH. This is why TSH levels are high when thyroid hormone levels are low and TSH is decreased when thyroid hormone levels are high.

The thyroid gland usually releases around 80 percent of its thyroid hormone as T4 and 20 percent as T3. Only 0.03 percent of the total T4 traveling around in the bloodstream is in the free form, in which it can be taken up into each body cell and do the job of effective thyroid hormone. Once the free T4 passes into a body cell of any kind, it is changed into T3 by an enzyme called 5-prime deiodinase.

Once changed, this T3 is absorbed into the nucleus of the cell, where the chromosomes are found. Inside the nucleus are special T3-receptor proteins that are made to stick to distinct spots in the genes of the chromosomes and also to stick to T3. When enough T3 is taken into the nucleus, it sticks to these T3-receptors and controls the genes that they are attached to. Some genes are turned on while other genes are turned off. Thus, each cell is able to convert the correct proportion of T4 to T3 for its own needs.

Be Informed:
Know the Facts About T4/T3

Many Internet sites and books falsely state that many people cannot convert T4 into T3. Converting T4 into T3 is necessary for life, and there is no evidence that this metabolic derangement can be acquired later in life. Anyone who could not convert T4 into T3 would not be alive, as this conversion is necessary for fetal development and birth.

This myth leads patients into potentially dangerous decisions about their treatment and into purchasing thyroid "support products" or T3 that they may not need. For information on how T3 levels are determined by measuring levels of the thyroid-stimulating hormone (TSH), see page 20.

The T4/T3 conversion myth is also used to support other false statements. One is that TSH tests can read as normal when you're really hypothyroid (this is false except for rare people with pituitary tumors). Another falsity is that dessicated pig thyroid hormone (sold as "natural" thyroid hormone), questionable herbal concoctions that "help" with T4/T3 conversion, or regular and chronic T3 supplementation is preferable to, or healthier than, taking levothyroxine alone at the appropriate dose.

Yang's Story: Damaged by the T4/T3 Conversion Myth

When I was diagnosed with hypothyroidism, I searched the Internet and read that people who do not properly convert T4 to T3 should avoid synthetic T4 [levothyroxine]. The website suggested that natural thyroid hormone from animals, which contained both T4 and T3, was preferable. After reading this, I didn't want to risk not converting my T3 properly and decided that the animal thyroid hormone was the best route for me.

My endocrinologist refused to give me animal thyroid hormone, so I followed the website's advice and went to see a holistic doctor (there was a list of them I clicked on). This doctor put me on a brand of pig thyroid hormone. None of this was covered by my health insurance because the holistic doctor did not accept insurance. At first I felt OK, but then I started to feel heart palpitations and all "speedy." My periods got very strange too. This went up and down for many months; at times I would feel normal, and then the palpitations would start up again. The holistic doctor I saw did not do any blood tests but prescribed some herbs that he said would help with "thyroid support." It took a long time for me to realize that I was being led astray.

Finally, I went to see another endocrinologist, who was wonderful and told me that she had many patients like me who read "some things on the Internet" that were not correct. I wasted about a year and a half with the wrong doctor taking the wrong pills. I later learned that the pig thyroid hormone had made me feel speedy because of too much T3—I was overdosed. I was very upset with myself for not questioning more about what I was reading. I thought that since I am well educated, I was able to navigate the Internet, but the health information is confusing.

Be Informed:
The Truth About Reverse T3

Many websites and books say that trauma and stress can create a "fake" normal T3 level, called reverse T3. The claim is that many people with so-called normal TSH levels really have reverse T3 and are actually hypothyroid. This theory takes fact and creates fiction.

T4 is converted to T3 by removing a specific iodine atom from each of the T4 molecules. If a different iodine is removed, reverse T3 is formed. Reverse T3 is inactive; it cannot do the job of T3 and therefore will not suppress TSH. It will not affect TSH levels at all. If T4 is converted to reverse T3 without making enough regular T3, your TSH levels will be high and you will be hypothyroid. If the TSH levels are normal, so are the levels of regular T3 inside of your cells.

The Role of Iodine in the Diet

T4 and T3, as already noted, are so named because of the number of iodine atoms per hormone molecule. So what is the role of iodine in the production of thyroid hormone? The thyroid gland needs to import one key ingredient for thyroid hormone production: iodine. Your thyroid gland extracts iodine from various foods, including fish, egg yolks, shellfish, milk products, and anything with iodized salt. Normally you take in sufficient iodine through your diet.

Thyroid glands are very sensitive to iodine. When the thyroid gland is not able to obtain sufficient quantities of iodine, you can develop a goiter, or an enlarged thyroid gland. A goiter can also develop if your thyroid gland is stimulated to take up too much iodine and produces too much thyroid hormone. Although it seems odd that too much or too little iodine can produce the same results, the reason the goiter develops in each case is different. The role iodine plays in the diet as well as the consequences of iodine deficiency are discussed more in Chapter 11.

The Role of the Pituitary Gland and Thyroid-Stimulating Hormone

The pituitary gland is situated at the base of the skull and is, without question, the most influential gland in your body. It is often referred to as the master gland. The pituitary gland acts as the body's "thermostat" by sending out many types of stimulating hormones to the various parts of our bodies that make hormones.

Your thyroid gland reports directly to the pituitary gland, which monitors T4 and T3 levels in your body. When levels are low, it secretes TSH; this signals the thyroid gland to make thyroid hormone. The TSH stimulates the thyroid to take up iodine from the blood and make thyroid hormone, just as a thermostat's electrical signal to the furnace stimulates it to take up fuel and make heat. When the thyroid hormone level in the blood rises to the proper level, it causes the pituitary to reduce its release of TSH, just as a thermostat turns off its electrical signal to the furnace. This regulates the thyroid hormone in the blood so that it stays at the proper level, in the same way the thermostat keeps a house at the proper temperature.

If the pituitary gland is working properly, a high level of TSH means that there is not enough thyroid hormone in the blood; a low level of TSH means that there is too high a level of thyroid hormone in the blood; and a normal level of thyroid hormone results in a normal level of TSH. The TSH level in the blood can be measured to tell whether the thyroid is making enough, too little, or too much thyroid hormone. The TSH test is the most accurate and sensitive blood test that exists for thyroid patients.

The Role of the Hypothalamus

The hypothalamus is a part of the brain located just above the pituitary gland. It is connected to the pituitary by a thin stalk that carries hormones that help control the pituitary. A part of the hypothalamus also works like a thyroid hormone thermostat, releasing its own signal, thyrotropin-releasing hormone (TRH), or TSH-releasing hormone, to the pituitary when the thyroid hormone levels are low. Thus there is a "double-thermostat" control of thyroid hormone in the body, although this can break down when something is wrong with the hypothalamus.

The Role of Calcitonin

In the thyroid gland, the cells that produce thyroid hormone are called follicular cells. Thyroid follicles are contained within the capsule of the thyroid gland like bunches of microscopic grapes. Between neighboring thyroid follicles are tiny blood vessels, lymph vessels, and collections of other cells, called parafollicular cells. These parafollicular cells, or C-cells, make additional hormones, such as calcitonin and somatostatin.

Calcitonin helps to regulate calcium and therefore helps to prevent osteoporosis. But to your bones, calcitonin is kind of like a tonsil. It serves a useful purpose, but when the hormone is not manufactured due to the absence of a thyroid gland (if it's removed or ablated by radioactive iodine), you won't really notice any effects, just as you don't miss your tonsils. Calcium levels are really controlled by the parathyroid glands and are much more dependent on Vitamin D, which helps with calcium absorption; diet; and exercise, which builds bone mass.

Calcitonin is only important when discussing the thyroid in the context of a rare type of thyroid cancer known as medullary thyroid cancer (see Chapter 6). When this type of thyroid cancer develops, your thyroid overproduces calcitonin, which is a marker for medullary thyroid cancer.

A Few Words About the Parathyroid Glands

There are usually four (though sometimes three to six) other glands located very close to the thyroid gland; they are called parathyroid glands, which literally means "near the thyroid." These glands do not produce thyroid hormone but instead make parathyroid hormone (PTH), which is important for controlling calcium in the body. It causes the kidneys to retain calcium in the blood while releasing phosphorus into the urine. At the same time, it increases the activation of vitamin D, which enhances the absorption of calcium and phosphorus from food and beverages.

These glands are sometimes damaged or accidentally removed during surgery on the thyroid gland. Although only one functioning parathyroid gland is needed, loss or damage to all four glands results in loss of parathyroid hormone, which reduces the absorption of calcium, causing calcium levels in the blood to fall. The symptoms of low calcium include muscle cramps and spasms, numbness, and, in severe cases, seizures. Likewise, losing the parathyroid glands causes phosphorus levels to stay high because the kidneys are not able to release it into the urine.

Damage to the parathyroid glands is a known risk of thyroid surgery. This risk is higher, however, when the surgeon is less experienced, when there is a need for multiple neck surgeries, or when a thyroid cancer is particularly invasive.

The Role of Thyroglobulin

Although this sounds like a Halloween candy, thyroglobulin (Tg) is a specific protein made only by your thyroid cells and is used mostly by the thyroid gland itself to make thyroid hormone. The only role thyroglobulin plays in the treatment of thyroid disease is as a screening marker for thyroid cancer recurrence. After your thyroid gland is removed as a consequence of any type of thyroid cancer (see Chapter 6), the protein thyroglobulin should not be manufactured anymore. If thyroglobulin is detectable on a blood test, it's a sign that some thyroid tissue remains, which could indicate a recurrence of thyroid cancer. Screening for thyroglobulin is useless for all other forms of thyroid disease.

Thyroid Disorders and Treatments: An Overview

The following is a summary of the most common thyroid disorders and their treatments, which will serve as a map to the rest of the book.

Hypothyroidism

Hypothyroidism is an underactive thyroid gland. If your thyroid gland is underactive and manufactures too little hormone, your bodily functions slow down. You'll have an unusually slow pulse, you'll feel very tired, and you'll have no energy. In addition, you might be constipated, you might get a little puffy, you might feel cold all the time, and your skin might get very dry. The most common cause of hypothyroidism is Hashimoto's thyroiditis, an autoimmune thyroid disease. Another common cause is aging; people over age sixty are vulnerable to mild hypothyroidism, which can be easily masked as fatigue associated with aging. See Chapter 2 for more details on hypothyroidism.

Hyperthyroidism

Hyperthyroidism is an overactive thyroid gland. If your thyroid gland is overactive and manufactures too much thyroid hormone, you will become thyrotoxic—toxic from too much thyroid hormone—and your body/heart rate will speed up. You might also feel hot all the time, have diarrhea, lose weight, and feel dizzy or shaky. This is known as thyrotoxicosis, discussed at length in Chapter 3. Hyperthyroidism is a common cause of thyrotoxicosis, but there are other causes as well. The most common is Graves' disease, an autoimmune thyroid disease that causes hyperthyroidism, which then causes thyrotoxicosis.

Another common cause of thyrotoxicosis is taking too much thyroid hormone, taking an unstable formulation of thyroid hormone (as in animal thyroid hormone), or taking T3 supplements (usually unnecessarily). Hyperthyroidism is discussed more in Chapter 3.

Thyroiditis

Thyroiditis is inflammation of the thyroid gland. Depending on what kind of thyroiditis you have, a goiter and symptoms of thyrotoxicosis or hypothyroidism can develop. Hashimoto's thyroiditis is an autoimmune disorder (see Chapter 2). The flulike de Quervain's thyroiditis, silent thyroiditis, and postpartum thyroiditis are usually temporary in nature. Acute suppurative thyroiditis is a bacterial thyroiditis usually seen in children. And Riedel's thyroiditis is caused by scar tissue. These forms of thyroiditis are discussed in Chapter 4.

Goiter

A goiter is an enlarged thyroid gland, and it is a sign that you may be hypothyroid or hyperthyroid. In previous generations, goiters were the way thyroid disorders were usually diagnosed; the appearance of the goiter was the telltale sign. Today, sensitive assay tests such as the TSH can usually diagnose thyroid diseases early, before the goiter appears. Goiters are discussed throughout the book, particularly in Chapters 2, 3, and 11.

Multinodular Goiter

A multinodular goiter is a bumpy or lumpy enlarged thyroid gland. For some unknown reason, one or more nodules, or lumps, form in your thyroid gland. These nodules can be "runaway trains" that mimic the thyroid gland, but they are not controlled by the thermostat system of the pituitary gland or the hypothalamus. The result is thyrotoxicosis. Many times, nodules do not make thyroid hormone. Ten percent of them turn out to be thyroid cancer. Nodules and multinodular goiters are discussed in Chapter 5.

Thyroid Cancer

Thyroid cancer is now the most quickly increasing type of cancer in both sexes and in all ages. There are several types of thyroid cancer, including follicular, papillary, and medullary. Treatments and follow-up care are discussed in Chapter 6.

Complications and Comorbidities

Thyroid disorders can affect other parts of your body. Thyroid eye disease, for example, is a condition marked by bulgy, watery eyes, frequently predates the diagnosis of Graves' disease. Cardiovascular diseases, sleep disorders and fatigue, and depression can all mask, complicate, or accompany thyroid disorders. And thyroid diseases can be aggravated by other factors, such as menopause or age. For the ins and outs of thyroid disease complications and comorbidities, see Chapter 7.

Thyroid Disease and New Life

Creating and bringing a new life into the world can be exciting. However, it can also bring on or complicate thyroid disorders. Infertility can be a result of thyroid disorders, while gestational hyperthyroidism and gestational hypothyroidism can also occur (gestational refers to during pregnancy). Women need to monitor their thyroid levels during pregnancy not only for their own sake, but also for their baby's healthy growth and development. Thyroid disorders in the context of fertility, pregnancy, and in newborns are discussed in Chapter 8.

Radioactive Iodine

Radioactive iodine (RAI) is used in scanning and treatment for a variety of thyroid disorders. Chapter 9 explains RAI usage for diagnostic tests, scans, and treatment and dispels misinformation about RAI. In addition, it discusses RAI scanning for people with thyroid cancer.

Thyroid Hormone Replacement Therapy

In most cases, the result of various thyroid diseases is that your thyroid gland will no longer make thyroid hormone at all, or in adequate amounts. When you are not making enough—or any—thyroid hormone, you need to find a way to replace it in your body. For more on thyroid hormone replacement, see Chapter 10.

Dietary Iodine and Other Diet-Related Issues

As discussed earlier, iodine is a necessary element for the proper functioning of the thyroid gland. Iodine deficiency can lead to goiters and, in newborns and young children, to mental deficiencies. There are times, however, when a low-iodine diet is necessary to prepare for an RAI scan or treatment. Dietary iodine, the low-iodine diet, and other diet- and weight-related issues are discussed in Chapter 11.

Complementary Therapies

Thyroid disorders and their treatments can affect the whole person, not just the thyroid gland. Complementary therapies—therapies that complement allopathic, or conventional medical, treatments—are discussed in Chapter 12.

2

Slowing Down

Hypothyroidism

HYPOTHYROIDISM IS ONE of the most common health problems in North America. If you are hypothyroid, it means that you don't have enough thyroid hormone in your body to function normally. Usually this is because the thyroid gland is underactive and is not making enough thyroid hormone for your body's requirements. Hypothyroidism can be mild, moderate, or severe. People most at risk for mild hypothyroidism are women, individuals over sixty, people with a family history of thyroid disease, or people with other autoimmune diseases, such as pernicious anemia, Type 1 diabetes, rheumatoid arthritis, or lupus.

Mild hypothyroidism affects 10 to 15 percent of all adults and 7 to 26 percent of people over sixty. It is more common in women than in men. In addition to developing primary hypothyroidism, anyone treated for a thyroid disorder will probably experience iatrogenic (treatment-caused) hypothyroidism at some point, because the treatments for other thyroid conditions usually result in hypothyroidism, quite deliberately and sometimes temporarily.

This chapter explains the symptoms of hypothyroidism, the most common causes of primary hypothyroidism, and treatment for hypothyroidism with thyroid hormone replacement. It also discusses the many conditions that can mimic or mask hypothyroidism, such as depression.

Symptoms of Hypothyroidism

When you are hypothyroid, everything in your body slows down, including your reflexes, your ability to maintain your body temperature, and your ability to respond to your environment. This slowing down occurs from head to toe; these symptoms are discussed here in alphabetical order. These symptoms disappear once your thyroid hormone level is restored to normal.

Cardiovascular Changes

People with hypothyroidism often have an unusually slow pulse rate (between forty and seventy beats per minute) and blood pressure that may be too high. More severe or prolonged hypothyroidism can raise your cholesterol levels as well, and this can aggravate blockage of your coronary arteries. In severe hypothyroidism, the heart muscle fibers may weaken, which can lead to heart failure. This scenario is rare, however, and you would have to suffer from severe and obvious hypothyroid symptoms for a long time before your heart would be at risk.

But even mild hypothyroidism may aggravate your risk for heart disease if you have other risk cofactors. For example, it's not unusual if you are hypothyroid to notice chest pain (which may be confused with angina) or shortness of breath when you exert yourself. You may notice some calf pain, which is caused by hardening of the arteries and dysfunction of the muscles in the leg. Fluid may also collect, causing your legs and feet to swell.

Cold Intolerance

Because your entire metabolic rate has slowed down, you may not be able to find a comfortable temperature. You may find yourself wondering, "Why is it always *freezing* in here?" You will likely carry a sweater with you all the time to compensate for your continuous sensitivity to cold. You'll feel much more comfortable in hot, muggy weather, and you may not even perspire in the heat.

Depression and Psychiatric Misdiagnosis

Hypothyroidism is linked to psychiatric depression more frequently than hyperthyroidism, but symptoms of depression may be masked or misdiagnosed in both cases (see Chapter 3 as well), and thus can cause the psychiatric misdiagnosis. Psychiatrists even find that hypothyroid patients sometimes exhibit certain behaviors linked to psychosis, such as paranoia or aural and visual hallucinations (hearing voices and seeing things that are not there). This used to be called "myxedema madness." Interestingly, in some populations roughly 15 percent of patients suffering from depression are found to be hypothyroid.

Digestive Changes and Weight Gain

Because your system has slowed down, you may suffer from constipation, hardening of your stools, bloating (which may cause bad breath), poor appetite, and heartburn. Food will not move through your stomach as quickly, so you may experience acid reflux (a condition in which semidigested food comes back up the esophagus). Because the lack of thyroid hormone slows down your metabolism, you might gain weight as well. But because your appetite may decrease radically, your weight could also stay the same.

Adonia's Story: Misdiagnosed as Depressed

When I was in my midforties, I started to have problems concentrating and wasn't really interested in much of anything. I thought I was perimenopausal, but my doctor diagnosed me with depression and put me on an antidepressant. This didn't really do anything other than make me lose complete interest in sex and gain weight. My hair started to fall out, and my doctor told me that this sometimes happens with antidepressants. I switched to another antidepressant, but I just couldn't seem to get better.

I was referred to an endocrinologist to see if I was menopausal, and he finally checked my thyroid. My TSH was about 35, which he told me meant I was severely hypothyroid. They gave me a drug, levothyroxine. Things began to improve. When I went off the antidepressant, my hair started to come back, and I was interested in sex again.

Hypothyroid patients can experience some, or all, of these symptoms. If the hypothyroidism is caught early enough, you may not be aware of any of these symptoms until your doctor asks if you have noticed specific changes.

You'll need to adjust your eating habits to compensate, which is discussed in more detail in Chapter 11. It is common to gain some weight over the course of two or more months when you are diagnosed with a hypothyroid condition, even though you may not be eating as much. Some of the weight gain, however, is due to bloating from constipation. The frequency of your bowel movements will decrease when you are hypothyroid and will usually improve after your thyroid hormone levels are restored to normal.

Enlarged Thyroid Gland

You may experience an enlarged thyroid gland, or goiter, either because it is scarred from Hashimoto's thyroiditis (see page 23) or from constant stimulation from high TSH levels. A goiter can also develop from Graves' disease, when too much thyroid hormone is produced (see Chapter 3).

Fatigue and Sleepiness

The classic symptom of hypothyroidism is a distinct, lethargic tiredness or sluggishness, causing you to feel unnaturally sleepy, even though you slept well for over twelve hours the night before. Your doctor may also notice that you exhibit delayed reflexes. Researchers now know that when you are hypothyroid, you are less able to reach Stage IV sleep, the deepest, most restful kind of sleep. Lack of restorative sleep partly explains why you feel tired, sleepy, and unrefreshed.

Fingernails

Your fingernails may become brittle and develop lines and grooves to the point where applying nail polish may be difficult.

Hair Changes

When you are hypothyroid, your hair may become thin, dry, and brittle, and you may find that you need additional hair conditioner. You may also lose some hair, to the point where it becomes sparse, or body hair, such as eyebrow, leg, arm, or pubic hair. Much of this grows back after some time on thyroid hormone replacement. If your thyroid hormone levels change over a short time, such as going from hypothyroidism to normal thyroid levels (euthyroidism), or from euthyroidism to hypothyroidism, you may experience transient increased hair loss, although your hair will grow back.

High Cholesterol

Hypothyroid patients often have high cholesterol, which can lead to a host of other problems, including heart disease. In fact, it's generally recommended that anyone with high cholesterol be tested for hypothyroidism. Your cholesterol level should be controlled through diet until your thyroid problem is brought under control. Cholesterol-lowering medications should not be started unless the high cholesterol levels persist for a few months after sufficient thyroid hormone replacement therapy.

Menstrual Cycle Changes

If you are female and hypothyroid, your menstrual periods will probably become much heavier and more frequent than usual. Your ovaries may even stop producing/releasing an egg each month. This can make conception difficult. You may also develop anemia resulting from these heavy periods.

Milky Discharge from Breasts

Hypothyroidism may cause you to overproduce prolactin, one of the hormones responsible for milk production. Too much prolactin can also block estrogen production, which will interfere with regular periods and ovulation. If you notice discharge coming out of your breast by itself and you are not lactating or deliberately expressing your breasts, get checked by a breast specialist or gynecologist (who should also perform a thorough breast exam to rule out other conditions).

Muscle Aches and Cramps

Hypothyroid patients commonly complain of muscle aches and cramps. Joints may also start to hurt. In fact, many people with hypothyroidism believe they are experiencing arthritic symptoms, although the condition completely clears up with thyroid hormone treatment. The aching can be severe enough to wake you up at night.

Muscle coordination can also be a problem. You may feel "klutzy" all the time and find it increasingly difficult to perform simple motor tasks. This clumsiness is a result of the effects of hypothyroidism on the coordination center in the brain.

Numbness

Numbness is combined with a sensation of "pins and needles." Hypothyroid patients also have a tendency to develop carpal tunnel syndrome, which is characterized by tingling and numbness in the hands. It is caused, in this case, by compression on nerves in the wrist due to thickening and swelling of the body tissues under the skin. This condition will usually resolve itself once your hypothyroidism is treated.

Poor Memory and Concentration

Hypothyroidism causes a "spacey" feeling, so you may find it difficult to remember things or to concentrate at work. This is especially scary for seniors, who may feel as though dementia is settling in. In fact, one of the most common causes of so-called "senility" is actually undiagnosed hypothyroidism.

Skin Changes

Your skin may feel dry and coarse to the point where it flakes like powder when you scratch it. Cracked skin can also become common

Be Informed:
Don't Drive While Hypothyroid

People who are moderately to severely hypothyroid, with TSH levels higher than 20, should not drive a vehicle of any kind, fly a plane, or operate heavy machinery. These rules do *not* apply to the vast majority of those who are mildly hypothyroid (usually with levels of 5 to 20). Thyroid cancer patients preparing for withdrawal scans (see Chapter 9), whose TSH levels typically go above 30 while in preparation, should definitely not drive while hypothyroid.

on your elbows and kneecaps. Your skin may develop a yellowish hue as the hypothyroidism worsens; this is caused by a buildup of carotene, a substance in our diet that is normally converted into vitamin A but slows its conversion due to hypothyroidism. Because your blood vessels are more tightly constricted, diverting blood away from your skin, you may also appear pale and washed out.

Other symptoms, which are more obvious to a physician, will be the presence of a condition known as myxedema, a thickening of skin and underlying tissues. Myxedema is characterized by puffiness around the eyes and face; it can even involve the tongue, which may swell.

Voice Changes

If your thyroid is enlarged, it may affect your vocal cords and cause your voice to sound hoarse or husky.

Diagnosing Hypothyroidism

The most important clue in diagnosing hypothyroidism is to look at the symptoms. People who have four or more of the symptoms of hypothyroidism outlined should be screened. It's more common for doctors to discover hypothyroidism before symptoms are obvious through a TSH test, which is done routinely during annual checkups.

Relying solely on symptoms without confirming through lab tests can be unreliable. If you surveyed a crowd about who was tired, overweight, constipated, or had dry skin, you would find that many people with normally functioning thyroid glands had those symptoms. The proper diagnostic tests will lead to a correct diagnosis. The two tests that correctly diagnose hypothyroidism are the free T4 test and the TSH test.

The Free T4 Test

To diagnose hypothyroidism, it's important that free T4 and not total T4 is measured. (The T3 level can be useful to assess thyroid hormone levels only in the case of thyrotoxicosis, not hypothyroidism.) This test provides useful information but cannot assess how the body "feels" in the same way as a TSH test. It is important to note that the laboratory tests for people with symptoms of hypothyroidism should include both a free T4 level and a TSH level because some people have a problem with their pituitary gland or brain that interferes with proper TSH production. In these situations, the free T4 level would be low while the TSH would be inappropriately normal or low.

The TSH Test

As discussed in Chapter 1, assessing TSH is by far the most valuable test for diagnosing thyroid disorder. Unfortunately, this test is also the most misunderstood by thyroid patients.

The most sensitive way to see how the body "feels" is to look at the body's natural "thermostat" for thyroid hormone, the pituitary gland. If the blood going to the pituitary gland (and the rest of the body) contains the proper amount of free T4, the level of TSH will be normal (0.5 to 4.0 mU/L). If you are hypothyroid, the TSH level will be higher than normal, since the pituitary seeks to stimulate your thyroid gland even if it isn't there or isn't working anymore. If you are thyrotoxic, the TSH level will be much lower than normal, since the pituitary will be attempting to diminish its stimulation of your thyroid gland.

Many laboratories might define their normal range for TSH as something close to 0.5 to 5.0; this is because years ago, the "normal" range was established through TSH tests on mostly men with "normal" thyroid glands—many of whom had mild hypothyroidism, which drove up the normal range for many years. This is partly what has spawned so much misinformation concerning the TSH test and caused patients to question its validity.

Knowledgeable physicians know that the true normal for most people is a range of 0.5 to 2.5. The American Association of Clinical Endocrinologists (AACE) revised its TSH targets in 2002, down to 0.3 to 3.0. Indeed, most people who are euthyroid sit between 0.4 and 2.5.

Revising the normal target to a more realistic range has helped many hypothyroid patients, women in particular, negotiate better care with their doctors. Newer targets also help to eliminate the hunt for bizarre (and incorrect) theories that attempt to explain why some people still feel hypothyroid when they are within the normal ranges. Most people will feel mild hypothyroid symptoms at numbers 10 or above. Mild or moderate hypothyroidism would show TSH levels ranging between 10 and 20, while severe hypothyroidism would be at levels above 30. TSH levels of less than 10 are in the range called early or subclinical hypothyroidism. Most people with TSH levels in this range do not have any symptoms that are clear signs of hypothyroid, but studies show they have subtle unhealthy changes in their bodies that are corrected when they take enough thyroid hormone to lower the TSH into the normal range. In addition, people with early hypothyroidism are at great risk of gradually becoming severely hypothyroid, so they should be started on thyroid hormone as soon as they are diagnosed.

Common Causes of Hypothyroidism

People who develop hypothyroidism as a primary condition due to the failure of the thyroid gland itself ("a broken thyroid") have primary hypothyroidism. This group includes people who develop thyroiditis from Hashimoto's disease or other causes, babies born without a thyroid gland, and people who have stopped making as much thyroid hormone as they used to due to aging. Congenital hypothyroidism is discussed in Chapter 8. In addition, iodine deficiency can lead to hypothyroidism (see Chapter 11).

People develop iatrogenic hypothyroidism as a result of having their thyroid glands surgically removed (see Chapter 6) or receiving

Be Informed:
The Truth About the TSH Test

Many websites and books mistakenly state that TSH tests are inaccurate and that use of this test is a sign that your doctor is not up to date. You may have read that the basal body temperature test (used in the 1930s) is more accurate or that it is best to just judge your thyroid hormone levels by the way you feel. All of this is untrue.

So long as your TSH levels are within the ranges discussed, the TSH test is very accurate for showing your thyroid hormone level to be sufficient. Basal body temperature testing has been discredited by all reliable patient thyroid organizations and professional associations, including the American Thyroid Association and all members of Thyroid Federation International (TFI). Many different factors unrelated to thyroid hormone affect the basal body temperature, as well as the basal metabolic rate (another type of test that has been promoted).

There are also pseudoscientific explanations about TSH levels that suggest that the test is inaccurate. One untrue statement is that "excess T3 generated at the pituitary level" can falsely suppress TSH, which is why TSH tests are not reliable in testing for hypothyroidism. Although this is an obviously false statement to anyone who understands basic medical science, it can sound true to those of us who are not scientists. As discussed in Chapter 1, T4 is converted into T3 by an enzyme called 5-prime deiodinase. This enzyme can be found in both the pituitary gland and the body's cells. No research has ever shown that the enzyme works differently in the pituitary than in body cells. The enzyme is what makes T3 out of T4, and therefore the TSH level accurately reflects the effect of thyroid hormones on the entire body.

radioactive iodine therapy for the purpose of ablating, or destroying, the thyroid gland (see Chapter 3). This is also considered primary hypothyroidism, because their thyroid glands no longer work, but these causes of hypothyroidism will not be discussed in this chapter.

Of note, roughly 25 to 50 percent of all people who have received external radiation therapy to the head and neck area for cancers such as Hodgkin's disease tend to develop hypothyroidism from thyroid gland failure within ten years of their treatment. It's recommended that people in this group have an annual TSH test.

Hashimoto's Thyroiditis

Thyroiditis means "inflammation of the thyroid gland." Hypothyroidism can develop from thyroiditis, and the most common cause of thyroiditis in North America is an autoimmune disease called Hashimoto's thyroiditis, or Hashimoto's disease. Other kinds of thyroiditis are discussed in Chapter 5.

In medical circles, Hashimoto's disease is referred to as chronic lymphocytic thyroiditis because it occurs when lymphocytes attack the thyroid gland. This disease is named after Hakaru Hashimoto, the Japanese physician who first described the condition in 1912. Like other autoimmune diseases, the tendency for Hashimoto's thyroiditis is inherited. Much of the time, Hashimoto's disease strikes adults over thirty (though many younger women have also been diagnosed with it), and it is much more frequently diagnosed in women than in men. Statistically, one in five women will probably develop Hashimoto's thyroiditis during her lifetime.

Hashimoto's disease is caused by abnormal autoantibodies and white blood cells that attack and damage thyroid cells. Eventually, this constant attack destroys many of the thyroid cells, and the absence of sufficient functional thyroid cells causes hypothyroidism. In most cases, a goiter develops because of the inflammation and overstimulation of the residual thyroid cells by TSH from the pituitary gland, although sometimes the thyroid gland shrinks instead.

If you develop Hashimoto's thyroiditis, you probably will not notice any symptoms at first. Sometimes there is a mild pressure in the thyroid gland and fatigue can set in, but unless you are on the lookout for thyroid disease because of your family history, Hashimoto's disease can go undetected for years. Only when the thyroid cells are damaged to the point that the thyroid gland functions inadequately will you begin to experience the symptoms of hypothyroidism.

Larissa's Story: The Hypothyroid Crash

After I had my first child, I couldn't seem to regain my energy. I thought it was just all the stress of coping with new motherhood. My doctor told me I had the "after-baby blues" and assured me it would pass. At first I noticed mostly tiredness, and then I started to have chronic constipation and a weird puffiness under my eyes. I just sort of dragged along and started to have problems concentrating. I felt horrible, like I was somehow a failure at being a mother.

One day when I was feeling very low, I called my mother and asked her if this was normal after a baby, and she remembered something she hadn't thought was important— that she had had a thyroid condition when I was born in the 1970s. When I went to my doctor two months later, she finally checked my thyroid. My doctor explained that I had Hashimoto's disease, which was why I was having all these symptoms. She prescribed thyroid hormone, and I started to feel better in about two weeks.

In rare instances, thyroid eye disease can set in as well (see Chapter 7). In many ways, Hashimoto's disease is the same as Graves' disease (see Chapter 3) except that the antibodies destroy the thyroid cells instead of stimulating the thyroid to make excessive thyroid hormone. In fact, the same antibodies seen in Hashimoto's disease are usually produced in Graves' disease as well. Treating eye problems associated with Hashimoto's disease involves treating the initial hypothyroidism first. If eye problems persist, the same treatment pattern outlined for Graves' disease will be necessary, as detailed in Chapter 7.

Rarer still, some people with Hashimoto's disease experience thyrotoxicosis *and* hypothyroidism. This occurs due to the two phases of the disease. First, the attack of the antibodies causes the stores of thyroid hormone within the thyroid gland to suddenly leak out, raising the thyroid hormone to a level in the blood that is too high. This condition is coined Hashitoxicosis. If you suffered from this somewhat paradoxical condition, you would first experience all the symptoms of thyrotoxicosis (see Chapter 3). After a month or two, the antibodies attacking the thyroid cells would cause them to stop working and the leaking stored hormones would be depleted, causing the thyrotoxicosis to resolve. Then, as the thyroid-destructive features of Hashimoto's disease progressed, you would eventually become hypothyroid, developing the symptoms of hypothyroidism.

Diagnosing Hashimoto's Thyroiditis

The signs of Hashimoto's disease are not at all obvious. In its early stages, a goiter can develop as a result of inflammation in the thyroid gland. The goiter is usually firm, but in rare cases can be tender. The goiter's presence can suggest Hashimoto's disease, but it is usually suspected because of the onset of symptoms of hypothyroidism. Age can be a factor in diagnosis as well, given that the disease is common in women over forty.

Hashimoto's disease is frequently missed as a diagnosis, however. Symptoms of hypothyroidism are often attributed to age, particularly in women entering menopause. Once suspected, Hashimoto's disease is easily diagnosed through a blood test that indicates high levels of thyroid autoantibodies called TPO (thyroid peroxidase) autoantibodies and antithyroglobulin (TG) antibodies in the blood. TSH levels must also be measured; high TSH levels indicate hypothyroidism and the need to take thyroid hormone medication.

Treating Hashimoto's Thyroiditis

The treatment for Hashimoto's disease is simple: thyroid hormone replacement is prescribed as soon as the diagnosis is made if TSH levels are high—even if there are no symptoms. Thyroid hormone suppresses production of excessive TSH by the pituitary gland, which, in turn, shrinks any goiter that may have developed or is about to develop. Also, because Hashimoto's disease often progresses to the point where clinical symptoms of hypothyroidism set in, the thyroid hormone prevents inevitable hypothyroidism. If you have developed a goiter as a result of Hashimoto's disease, the goiter will usually persist unless you take thyroid hormone. There might be so much scarring in the thyroid gland that the goiter never shrinks; in this case, you may want to have a thyroidectomy, or complete removal of the thyroid gland, if the goiter causes difficulty swallowing. After the thyroidectomy you would still need to take thyroid hormone. It takes anywhere from six to eighteen months for the goiter to shrink; if and when it does shrink, you will need to continue taking levothyroxine to treat your hypothyroidism.

Subclinical Hypothyroidism

Subclinical hypothyroidism, or mild hypothyroidism, refers to hypothyroidism that has not progressed very far, meaning that you have few or no symptoms as of now. The most common cause of this is Hashimoto's thyroiditis. On a blood test, your free T4 readings would be normal or very close to normal but your thyroid-stimulating hormone readings would be higher than normal.

If you meet any of the following criteria, you should be screened for subclinical hypothyroidism by having an annual TSH test.

- Anyone with a family history of thyroid disease
- Women planning pregnancy
- Pregnant women (very important!)
- Women who have just given birth (very important!)
- Women over forty
- Anyone over sixty
- Anyone with symptoms of depression, especially postpartum depression, or who has been diagnosed with depression
- Anyone with symptoms and/or a diagnosis of chronic fatigue syndrome or fibromyalgia
- Anyone newly diagnosed with PMS (premenstrual syndrome) or perimenopause symptoms
- Anyone diagnosed with premature menopause, early menopause, or premature ovarian failure
- Anyone with another autoimmune disease, especially rheumatoid arthritis, lupus, or Type 1 diabetes

Less Common Causes of Hypothyroidism

There are less common causes of hypothyroidism—which I will not elaborate on in this book given their rarity—that include:

- Certain drugs, such as lithium (see Chapter 10)
- Pituitary gland disorders
- Tumors or cysts on the pituitary gland
- Rare problems with the hypothalamus

Treating Hypothyroidism

Treating hypothyroidism involves taking thyroid hormone, which either replaces the thyroid hormone you're no longer making or supplements thyroid hormone to compensate for the inadequate amount your thyroid is making. What isn't so simple is finding the right dosage and restoring your thyroid levels to normal, as determined by the TSH test. Thyroid hormone—in all its formulations—is discussed in detail in Chapter 10.

There are rare cases when thyroid hormone doesn't work well, such as a rare genetic disorder called thyroid hormone resistance, of which only 350 cases are cited worldwide. Thyroid hormone also doesn't work if you don't take it properly; are taking medications or supplements that interfere with its absorption; or are taking pills inactivated by heat, which is a much bigger problem than you would think (see Chapter 10). People with celiac disease (or other absorption problems) may have problems with thyroid hormone absorption, too. In all cases where thyroid hormone doesn't work well, you will remain hypothyroid and have high TSH levels, which will be seen on a TSH test.

Feeling Hypothyroid When Your Tests Are Normal

If you have normal TSH levels but still have symptoms of hypothyroidism, then you should be relieved to know that the persistent symptoms are not likely to be related to your hypothyroidism and you can investigate other causes and remedies. The goal of treating hypothyroidism is to restore your thyroid levels to normal. The hypothyroid state in your body may exist along with other problems (see Chapter 7). Ask anyone who is not hypothyroid if they're tired, depressed, constipated, or achy,

Sujata: An Unusual Case of Graves' Disease

Just after my fortieth birthday, I started to lose a lot of weight without trying and then noticed that my heart was beating fast. Since I was already thin, I was not happy about losing weight, and my clothes stopped fitting me. Sometimes at night, my heart would be racing so fast that it would wake me up.

I went to the doctor, where I learned I was hyperthyroid and had Graves' disease. I was prescribed a medication to slow down my heart rate, and they told me that I should come back in a month or so to discuss the next steps. After a couple of weeks on the heart medication, I started to feel very unwell. I was very tired and took my own pulse and it was only about forty beats per minute, which seemed too slow. I thought I was on too high a dose of this drug and called my doctor. They took me off the drug and told me to see how I felt. Nothing changed, and I started to feel very tired and sort of "draggy."

I went to the doctor in another two weeks, as planned, and they did some more tests and told me that I had "a very unusual case of Graves' disease" because it disappeared. Now my thyroid was not working at all. They told me that it either "burned out" by itself, or I could have Hashitoxicosis, where I start off hyperthyroid and then become hypothyroid. My doctor prescribed levothyroxine, and I started to feel better soon.

and a huge majority will say yes to at least one of those complaints in spite of normal thyroid levels and no history of thyroid disease.

The Truth About Hidden Hypothyroidism

There are numerous false and bizarre theories about why hidden hypothyroidism persists in spite of normal TSH levels. It's important to understand that it's not really hidden hypothyroidism, but *hidden causes for your symptoms* that can mimic (or, in most cases, mask) hypothyroidism. In other words, you can continue to feel "hypothyroid" when you're not because the symptoms of hypothyroidism overlap with other causes not related to thyroid problems. These include physical and emotional stress; sleep deprivation; normal aging, including menopause; sedentary living; poor diet; obesity or obesity-related diseases, such as diabetes or cardiovascular disease; and many others. Remember, too, that bouts of hypothyroidism seriously interfere with your normal activities. Many people become more sedentary, gain weight, and consequently feel bad even after their thyroid hormone levels are restored. Bouts of hypothyroidism can leave you out of the loop at work and in your social life, and you may feel the consequences of catching up or the long absence of engagement in your community or your social network; in turn, that can trigger real depression.

It's important to understand that you can't blame all your symptoms of poor health on your thyroid condition, especially when you have cofactors for other diseases. This includes poor social support systems at home, which can predispose people to depression. In short, there are things going on in your life and body other than hypothyroidism; indeed, many people have multiple health conditions simultaneously.

Be Informed: Don't Believe These Myths About Hypothyroidism

Rumors and myths about hypothyroidism are a crowded area on the Internet and in many books. Here are the most common myths you may have read—and the truth behind them.

MYTH: *Thyroid hormone resistance is a common cause of hidden hypothyroidism.*

FACT: In the extremely rare genetic disorder called thyroid hormone resistance, or Refetoff Syndrome, much greater quantities of T4 are needed to activate the proper genes. This has been distorted on the Internet and in some books as a common disorder leading to persistent hypothyroidism despite normal TSH levels. This is completely false.

MYTH: *Hidden hypothyroidism is common.*

FACT: Many websites and books claim that the TSH test cannot detect hypothyroidism in many people and that low body temperature is the best way to measure hypothyroidism. These claims support false theories about so-called "hidden hypothyroidism" and ways to diagnose and treat it, using either natural thyroid hormone or T3 alone. This belief system has organized into two thyroid groups: Broda Barnes followers and Wilson's thyroid syndrome followers (see next two myths).

MYTH: *Broda O. Barnes's theories are valid.*

FACT: The theories springing from the ideas of late physician Broda O. Barnes go like this: Most people have hypothyroidism and don't know it, which is the underlying cause of almost all ill health in the Western world, from heart disease and diabetes to infections, from emphysema to cancer. According to Barnes, lab blood tests are completely inaccurate in testing for hypothyroidism. He advises that the best way to diagnose hypothyroidism is by measuring basal body temperature with a home thermometer. According to the Barnes method, if your morning temperature is below 97.8°F, then you are hypothyroid. This doesn't make sense when you consider that the normal body temperature, 98.7°F, was found to fluctuate wildly in many well-done studies published in the medical literature. The American Thyroid Association has an open warning about basal body temperature testing. Followers of Barnes believe that levothyroxine doesn't work, which is false. The "Barnes system" of self-diagnosing hypothyroidism can lead to someone who will sell you lots of other tests comprising a full metabolic workup. Dr. Barnes practiced medicine from the 1930s through the 1970s, in an era that predated modern TSH tests and refined formulations of levothyroxine. This is probably why Barnes's writings discuss outdated tests and treatments, which have been repackaged to thyroid patients as an alternative.

MYTH: *Wilson's thyroid syndrome is the cause of my hidden hypothyroidism.*

FACT: Wilson's syndrome is not a thyroid disease or condition recognized by any conventional thyroid practitioners or by the American Thyroid Association. Named by Dr. Denis E. Wilson, it borrows from some of Broda Barnes's theories about low body temperature as a sign of unrecognized hypothyroidism in spite of normal thyroid lab tests. Wilson also suggests that a host of nonspecific ill-health symptoms, which can be attributed to hundreds of conditions, combined with low body temperature, means you have Wilson's thyroid syndrome, which can only be treated with a special preparation of T3. There is simply no basis for this treatment, even if hypothyroidism *were* discovered, based on the strange diagnostic methods and criteria proposed in this theory. Biochemically, if you give someone with normal thyroid function T3 when they don't need it, they will become thyrotoxic, possibly leading to heart problems and even to death.

MYTH: *Experiencing weight gain despite normal TSH levels means you're hypothyroid.*

FACT: Many people struggle with their weight without any kind of thyroid problem. Sadly, being treated for hypothyroidism with thyroid hormone therapy does not automatically disqualify one from weight control issues. During bouts of untreated hypothyroidism, you may gain weight, similar to weight gain after childbirth or after a weeklong cruise with all-you-can-eat buffets. Just like women may have to work at getting rid of their pregnancy weight gain, you may have to work at getting rid of extra pounds put on before your hypothyroidism was treated. Chapter 11 discusses diet and thyroid disease in more detail.

3

Speeding Up

Thyrotoxicosis and Hyperthyroidism

MANY THYROID PATIENTS—and even doctors—confuse two distinct terms: *hyperthyroidism*, which means "overactive thyroid gland," and *thyrotoxicosis*, which means "too much thyroid hormone." Hyperthyroidism and thyrotoxicosis are cousins that often pass as twins. The overactive thyroid gland of hyperthyroidism classically causes too much thyroid hormone to be produced in your body. All the hyperthyroid symptoms you may have read about or heard about are, in fact, symptoms of too much thyroid hormone, which may indeed result from an overactive thyroid gland (hyperthyroid). But too much thyroid hormone can also result from other thyroid diseases—most commonly Graves' disease—as well as too high a dosage of thyroid hormone taken as a medication.

Signs of Thyrotoxicosis

The signs of hypothyroidism involve an overall slowing down (see Chapter 2). With hyperthyroidism, the opposite happens. When you have too much thyroid hormone in your body, everything speeds up. Numerous physical symptoms can result, which are discussed here alphabetically. The good news is that the vast majority of these symptoms disappear once the cause of thyrotoxicosis is treated and your thyroid hormone levels are restored to normal.

Adrenaline Rush

The hormones released by the adrenergic system are called catecholamines. Two of these hormones are adrenaline (epinephrine) and noradrenaline (norepinephrine). High levels of thyroid hormone make you much more sensitive to the effects of your own adrenaline. Consequently, when thyroid hormone levels increase, your heart beats very fast from the combined effects of both adrenaline and thyroid hormone. Medications called beta-blockers are useful to help slow the heart down and prevent severe heart symptoms that can make thyrotoxicosis dangerous. You may notice the rapid heartbeat in thyrotoxicosis, or you may not. You may only notice it at bedtime when you are lying quietly and trying to go to sleep, as relayed by Sujata's story in Chapter 2. Once in a while, it may be severe enough to cause a heart rhythm problem called atrial fibrillation.

Behavioral and Emotional Changes

Thyrotoxic people experience a range of emotional symptoms. Nervousness; restlessness, or the inability to sit quietly and calmly; anxiety; irritability; sleeplessness, or the inability to sustain sleep for long periods of time; and insomnia are common problems. A thyrotoxic person may exhibit some, all, or none of these symptoms; it depends on the individual.

Some thyrotoxic people are emotionally fickle and easily angered. Others may have disordered thoughts, sometimes severe enough to become frank paranoia. Some people have such severe behavioral problems that their thoughts become bizarre and delusional, although this is rare. This may warrant care by a psychiatrist until thyroid levels stabilize.

Psychiatric Misdiagnosis

Psychiatrists see so many thyroid patients who have been referred to them as "psychiatric" patients that thyroid function tests have now become standard medical practice for most psychiatric referrals.

When people experience the exhaustion of too much thyroid hormone and the natural anxiety that accompanies it, but they do not notice or report other physical manifestations such as a fast pulse or too-frequent bowel movements (which can also be attributed to anxiety), they are often misdiagnosed with anxiety or panic disorders.

Depression, which is more typically masked by, or confused with hypothyroidism (see Chapter 2), can also be masked by, or confused with hyperthyroidism. It can manifest with irritability, sadness, poor appetite, weight loss, sleeplessness, lack of energy, lack of sex drive, anxiety, and panic. Thyrotoxic symptoms unfortunately mimic these same manifestations. Finally, thyrotoxicosis can sometimes cause euphoric mood swings, a characteristic of a mania, which is present in bipolar disorder.

Alethea's Story: High Anxiety or Hyperthyroidism?

I am apparently one of those post-9/11 Graves' patients, as I understand a whole bunch of us were diagnosed in the aftermath, since autoimmune disorders can be stress induced. I work in Manhattan and was really affected for months after 9/11. I started to suffer from what I thought was anxiety. I was diagnosed by my family doctor with generalized anxiety disorder (GAD). I worried a lot about many things—it was like a disease that I couldn't get any relief from. My doctor explained to me that when a worry persists for no logical reason and there is no relief, this is anxiety. It interfered with my job. I had a sense of dread and this constant "fright" about my personal safety. I walked around with heart palpitations, had problems sleeping, and lost a lot of weight. This went on for a long time, and then I noticed one day that my throat was sort of bulging, and my doctor looked at it and said, "Oh—that's your thyroid. You may have hyperthyroidism." She took some tests and I was diagnosed with Graves' disease. I was put on a beta-blocker and an antithyroid medication, which alleviated my symptoms.

Unfortunately, women especially may suffer from continuous and classic psychiatric misdiagnoses. One reason is that thyroid disorders occur much more frequently in women. Another reason is that thyrotoxic symptoms can mimic either depression or bipolar disorder, both diagnosed in women more frequently than men. Partly because of unfair social arrangements, where women still do "double-duty" or are marginalized and because women will seek help more often than men, women are treated for depression, anxiety, and bipolar disorder more often than men, and thyrotoxicosis may be missed.

Bowel Movements

More frequent bowel movements, or "hyperdefecation," is another sign of thyrotoxicosis. This is different than diarrhea because the bowel movements will not be liquidlike but appear to be normal. They'll just occur more often—even if your diet is normal and hasn't changed. Because your digestion speeds up, so do your bowels. Sometimes the buildup of thyroid hormone will prevent your small intestine from absorbing certain nutrients from food as well. If you suffered from chronic constipation prior to your thyroid problem, you may simply notice regularity naturally happens without laxatives or fiber. You may even notice that you have magically lost seven to ten pounds, although you have been eating more than usual.

Easy Bruising

Because some common platelet disorders are caused by autoimmunity, and people with one autoimmune disease are likely to have another one, these disorders can occur with autoimmune thyroid disease. Platelet disorders may cause increased bruising. Aspirin can make the bruising worse. Easy bruising can also occur without associated platelet problems, because capillaries (very small blood vessels) are made more fragile by thyrotoxicosis.

Enlarged Thyroid Gland

As discussed in Chapter 1, an enlarged thyroid gland, called a goiter, is what happens when your thyroid enlarges and swells in the front of your neck. Thyrotoxic goiters develop due to hyperthyroidism—

too much stimulation of the thyroid causes the gland to enlarge. In extreme cases, a goiter can swell to the diameter of a grapefruit, but it is usually the size of a plum.

Eye Problems

Eye changes seen with thyrotoxicosis are related to the adrenergic effects already discussed, which cause the eyelid to retract. This is often called the *thyroid stare*. Additional eye changes, called *Graves' ophthalmopathy* or *thyroid eye disease (TED)*, frequently accompany Graves' disease. The muscles surrounding the eyeball swell, causing the eyeball to protrude (proptosis). In addition, the skin around the eyes swells (periorbital edema) and the whites of the eyes become red and irritated. This is discussed more in Chapter 7.

Exhaustion

When your body is overworked as a result of too much thyroid hormone, this can lead to exhaustion, which will affect your energy level and your general emotional well-being. Difficulty sleeping and sleep deprivation may be partly to blame. Weak muscles, discussed later, are another factor. Although you may have read online or elsewhere that increased levels of thyroid hormone give you more energy, the opposite is much more common.

Fingertip and Fingernail Changes

Some thyrotoxic people notice that their fingertips are swollen to the point where they look clubbed. This is known as *acropachy*, or clubbing. Fingernail growth also increases, but the nails become soft and easy to tear off. In addition, an alarming condition known as *onycholysis* can occur in which the upper edge of the fingernail becomes partially separated from the fingertip.

Hair Changes

Hair often becomes softer and finer in thyrotoxicosis patients and may not be as easy to style as it once was. Curly hair tends to become straighter. In some cases, you may notice some hair loss and find clumps of it on your pillow, clothing, tub, or hairbrush. This usually happens when there are big changes in your thyroid hormone levels. Your hair may also become grayer and may not "take" perms or color. There could be a general thinning of your hair, but once your thyroid hormone levels are restored to normal, your hair should grow as it once did. To create less stress on your hair, you should avoid coloring or perms until your hair follicles are stronger.

Heat Intolerance

A classic sign of thyrotoxicosis is intolerance to heat. Your body temperature may rise a bit; however, even normal room temperatures will feel too warm. In addition, you will sweat far more than usual. This combination is unpleasant, and you are likely to feel isolated in your discomfort. Typically, someone who is thyrotoxic is constantly wondering: "Is it me, or is it really hot in here?" Because this symptom mimics the hot flashes of menopause, thyrotoxicosis is often missed in women approaching menopause.

Heart Palpitations

One of the first signs of thyrotoxicosis is a rapid, forceful heartbeat. Increased levels of thyroxine released from the thyroid gland stimulate the heart to beat faster and stronger. In addition, thyrotoxicosis makes you more sensitive to your own adrenaline, further stimulating your heart rate. You will not notice an increase in your heart rate until it becomes severe. When a heartbeat is noticeably fast (sometimes as high as 150 beats per minute), and you are conscious of it beating in your chest, you are experiencing a palpitation. Thyrotoxic individuals often notice palpitations when they are reading, sleeping, or involved in other relaxing activities.

Once your thyroid hormone levels are restored to normal, your heart will resume its normal rate. But untreated palpitations can lead to serious heart problems. You may experience atrial fibrillation, a common heart rhythm abnormality, although this symptom is rare in thyroid patients. This means that your heart may have an irregular heart rhythm with random pauses and bursts of heartbeats. This condition is serious and is often associated with some degree of underlying heart disease; it should be treated by a cardiologist (heart specialist).

Another problem with a fast pulse is that it may create congestive heart failure, which can cause swollen ankles and even a collection of fluid in the chest. Shortness of breath may also develop, particularly if you are over sixty-five or have underlying heart problems. For this reason, it is not unusual for hyperthyroidism to be misdiagnosed as asthma, bronchitis, or heart disease.

Thyroid-related heart problems are treated with beta-blockers that slow the heart down (see page 55). This is often the first medication prescribed, because you need to block the effect of thyrotoxicosis on the heart, preventing the high thyroid hormone levels from over-stimulating the heart and possibly causing cardiovascular disease.

Infertility

Too much thyroid hormone can interfere with a woman's ovulation cycle, resulting in temporary infertility. Once thyroid hormone levels are restored to normal, in the absence of other barriers (e.g., endometriosis or blocked tubes), fertility is restored.

Thyrotoxicosis in early pregnancy can lead to miscarriage; repeated miscarriage is often considered a form of infertility. If this is a problem for you, it's important to insist that your TSH levels are checked to rule out an underlying thyroid problem. See Chapter 8 for more details.

Low Blood Sugar

Low blood sugar, also known as hypoglycemia, triggers the very same adrenaline-rush reaction that can occur during a panic attack. Officially, low blood sugar can be measured, and a reading below 50 mg/dl (3.5 mmol/L) is considered too low. But many people assume they suffer from low blood sugar even when their blood sugar levels are normal because they feel shaky and irritable when hungry, and the shakiness is relieved by food.

In fact, the common feature of panic attacks and true hypoglycemic attacks is a rapid activation of the adrenergic system, the same system enhanced by thyrotoxicosis. In this way, thyrotoxicosis can be mistaken for both panic attacks and false episodes of hypoglycemia. Treatment of these adrenergic symptoms by beta-blockers can relieve most of these symptoms, and correction of the underlying thyrotoxicosis relieves the rest of them.

Menstrual Cycle Changes

Thyrotoxic women will find that their periods are lighter and scanter, and they may even skip periods. Because thyroid problems interfere with ovulation and regular cycles, they also affect fertility. When thyroid hormone levels are restored to normal, cycles should return to normal.

Muscle Weakness

Muscle weakness is common in thyrotoxicosis and is especially noticeable in the shoulders, hips, and thighs, which can make it difficult to climb stairs. Your thigh muscles may in fact ache or feel soft. Shoulder weakness is noticed when you brush your hair or perform upper arm movements for long periods of time. Muscle symptoms are greatly exacerbated by worsening of arthritis or osteoporosis. Muscle weakness may be due partly to an overworked, exhausted body; however, there is good reason to believe that thyrotoxicosis has a direct effect on muscle function, sometimes causing wasting of skeletal muscles. If you have this muscle weakness, it's important to rule out another common autoimmune disease, myasthenia gravis, which afflicts muscles, causing profound weakness.

Sexual Function and Libido

Thyrotoxic men can experience a decreased libido, which seems to be related to increased signs of estrogen effects, including abnormally enlarged breasts. Some of this may be because thyrotoxicosis increases the amount of sex hormone–binding globulin, or protein, made by the liver, reducing the amount of testosterone available to enter body cells. Men with hyperthyroidism may complain of impotence. Some men may also experience low sperm count and thus impaired fertility. If a young adolescent male develops hyperthyroidism, he may experience a delay in development during normal puberty. Some men do not seem to have any negative effects on their libido during thyrotoxicosis. Of course, the complex effects of thyrotoxicosis on brain function, which alter thoughts and behavior, might have additional and differing effects on libido.

The effects of thyrotoxicosis on women's sexuality are unclear. Some women may have an increased desire for sex because of the effects of thyrotoxicosis on brain function and behavior. On the other hand, thyrotoxicosis-associated weakness and menstrual irregularities may combine to reduce a woman's sense of well-being and sex drive.

Skin Changes

Thyrotoxicosis may cause your skin to develop a fine, silky texture and to feel moist with remarkably few wrinkles. Because of enhanced perspiration, the constant moisture may cause a rash from inflamed pores. You may have areas of the skin that darken, particularly in the creases of your palms, and areas that become abraded or areas that itch. Your skin may even become sensitive to touch, swelling with minimal contact so that you can seemingly write your name on your skin.

Tremors

Trembling hands are one of the classic signs of thyrotoxicosis. You may notice that you have a tremor, meaning that you feel a little nervous and shaky all the time. This is a part of the adrenalinelike effect of thyrotoxicosis discussed earlier in this chapter. It can improve when your levels of thyroid hormone are restored to normal or when you take a beta-blocker.

Weight Loss

Sometimes the increased bowel activity associated with thyrotoxicosis, combined with an increased metabolic rate, contributes to weight loss—in spite of a healthy appetite. Overweight thyrotoxic people find this an unexpected bonus. It is this single tendency, however, that is responsible for a misunderstanding of thyroid and weight issues and for the misuse of thyroid hormone as a weight-loss drug (see Chapter 11 for more details on weight).

Weight loss is usually limited to ten to twenty pounds, and not all patients necessarily lose weight. Thyrotoxicosis often causes severe exhaustion, and some patients end up gaining weight because they become less active and their appetite is stimulated by their thyrotoxicosis.

"Thyroid Storm"

In some cases, symptoms of severe thyrotoxicosis can manifest as a "storm" of severe thyrotoxic symptoms—particularly cardiovascular symptoms that warrant emergency attention and admission to an intensive care unit. This used to happen more frequently, but since the use of beta-blockers and the development of the TSH test, as well as more active screening for subclinical thyrotoxicosis (before serious or noticeable symptoms develop), it is unusual for people with thyrotoxicosis to progress to such severe symptoms.

There is no intrinsic difference between the thyroid hormone levels in people with severe thyrotoxicosis with or without thyroid storm. The main difference is the effects on their bodies, particularly their hearts, and whether their heart rate is due to excessive thyroid hormone levels. Changes in medical management, including the introduction of beta-blockers, have significantly reduced the number of people with thyroid storm, to the point that it is now an exceedingly rare diagnosis.

Maria's Story: Panic Attacks or Thyroid Disorder?

When I was finishing my nursing degree, I started to suffer from panic attacks. They grew so extreme that I worried I would be caught in public with an attack and became afraid to leave my house. I would get a racing pulse, and then it would fade to a sort of fluttery heartbeat. Then I'd get this cold sweat and extreme vertigo—dizzy, nauseated, shaky. A couple of times I fainted in public. Every time it would happen, I would feel not in my body—like I was in a nightmare or dream. There was a sense of doom that would come over me. I finally went to my doctor about this, and they took a bunch of tests. My thyroid test was abnormally low, and I was diagnosed with Graves' disease. I was given a beta-blocker and the symptoms and panic attacks went away.

Graves' Disease: The Most Common Cause of Hyperthyroidism

About 80 percent of all hyperthyroidism is caused by Graves' disease, an autoimmune thyroid disease. Graves' disease is the next most common autoimmune thyroid disease after Hashimoto's thyroiditis (see Chapter 2). It is named after Robert James Graves, the nineteenth-century Irish physician who published a description of three patients with this condition in 1835 in the *London Medical and Surgical Journal*. Graves' disease occurs in both sexes and at all ages. It tends to affect women, usually between the ages of twenty and forty, individuals in their fifties or sixties, and young children. Similar to Hashimoto's disease, Graves' disease occurs much more frequently in women than men. Even so, roughly 1 percent of the population has Graves' disease, including former U.S. President George H. W. Bush, former First Lady Barbara Bush, and even their dog! The late John F. Kennedy Jr. suffered from Graves' disease as well.

How Graves' Disease Works

Graves' disease is a condition in which an abnormal antibody called thyroid-stimulating antibody (TSA) or thyroid-stimulating immunoglobulin (TSI) is produced. TSA stimulates the thyroid gland to vastly overproduce thyroid hormone. Normally controlled by the pituitary gland, the thyroid's triggers are tricked into being stimulated by abnormal antibodies. The result is hyperthyroidism. A goiter frequently develops, although it may be so minimal that your doctor cannot feel it.

The symptoms of Graves' disease are those of thyrotoxicosis, which were previously discussed. But there are some additional, unique complications, which may include the following.

• **Thyroid eye disease (TED).** Also called Graves' ophthalmopathy (GO) or Graves' orbitopathy, thyroid eye disease can be quite severe in people with Graves' disease (see Chapter 7). The majority of thyrotoxic Graves' disease patients suffer from measurable TED.

• **Heart disease risks.** The racing heart that is characteristic of thyrotoxicosis can complicate preexisting heart disease or worsen risk factors that predispose you to heart disease, even in the absence of Graves' disease. This is discussed further in Chapter 7.

• **Diabetes complications.** Thyrotoxicosis can increase your need for insulin if you have Type 1 diabetes or, in some cases, Type 2 diabetes. If you have Type 2 diabetes, you are already at a much greater risk of heart attack or stroke because of blood vessel complications. It is critical that you have your diabetes medications or insulin and your blood sugar targets reassessed by your doctor, as they can be thrown off by the symptoms of Graves' disease and thyrotoxicosis. If you have diabetic eye disease, it's important to assess whether any new eye symptoms are a result of developing thyroid disease or a worsening of preexisting diabetes eye disease.

• **Loss of pigmentation (vitiligo).** Vitiligo is an autoimmune attack on melanin-containing skin cells that may affect people with Graves' disease. Likewise, some people with Graves' disease develop a thickening of the skin over the lower legs called *pretibial myxedema.* The skin becomes firm and swollen and slightly darker in color. This is thought to be a reaction to the autoimmune antibodies of Graves' disease and is sometimes treated with steroid creams or ointments. In some cases the skin under the fingernails becomes remarkably thick, causing the ends of the fingers to thicken. In addition, loss of hair from autoimmune disease may be permanent and can result in baldness over the entire body.

Diagnosing Graves' Disease

The signs of Graves' disease are often obvious: you may develop a goiter and display all the classic signs of thyrotoxicosis. Or you may just develop symptoms of thyroid eye disease, which are usually telltale signs of Graves' disease. When the signs are obvious, your doctor simply confirms the diagnosis with blood tests that check your thyroid hormone levels and sometimes tests for the presence of antithyroid antibodies in the blood.

If you suspect that you have Graves' disease because it runs in your family or you're experiencing subtle symptoms, it can be detected through blood tests that check thyroid function, which include free T4, free T3, and TSH tests (see Chapter 2). If your thyroid function tests confirm hyperthyroidism, your doctor will look for evidence of associated autoimmune symptoms, such as Graves' ophthalmopathy or skin changes. Your physician will also try to establish a historical record of symptoms to see how long you have had symptoms of thyrotoxicosis. Long-term thyrotoxic symptoms make it less likely that transient thyroiditis is the cause of the thyrotoxicosis.

If the symptoms of hyperthyroidism or thyrotoxicosis are not obvious, a radioactive iodine uptake scan (see Chapter 9) will show increased thyroid gland radioactive iodine uptake in Graves' disease and little or no absorption in thyroiditis.

Sometimes, a blood test to measure TSA levels may prove useful. Since Graves' disease is responsible for 80 percent of all cases of thyrotoxicosis in those without a previous history of thyroid disease, most physicians routinely screen for it when thyrotoxicosis is diagnosed. If Graves' disease is not obvious or there is a lumpy gland, a radioactive iodine scan (see Chapter 9) may be needed to make the diagnosis and exclude thyroid nodules (see Chapter 5).

Treating Graves' Disease

There is no way to treat the root cause of Graves' disease—the autoimmune disorder itself. Therefore, treating Graves' disease involves treating hyperthyroidism. There are several distinctly different treatment methods, each with their own advantages and disadvantages. To treat hyperthyroidism, the thyroid gland is either rendered inactive and purposely destroyed with radioactive iodine (see Chapter 9) or surgically removed through a thyroidectomy (see Chapter 6). The goal of either therapy is to make you deliberately hypothyroid; it will then be necessary for you to receive thyroid hormone treatment for life. Graves' disease will cause your thyroid gland to burn out naturally anyway; therapy speeds up the process so you don't have to exist in a long-term state of thyrotoxicosis. Alternatively, you can be treated with antithyroid medication (discussed in an upcoming section), which in some (usually mild) cases, can lead to remission, meaning you can stop taking the medication because you are back to normal thyroid hormone levels.

It is important to realize that hypothyroidism is the goal of therapy. There is a great deal of incorrect material available concerning Graves' disease. One myth is that hypothyroidism is a sign that you received too high a dose of radioactive iodine *or* too much of your thyroid gland was removed. This is not true. There is also misinformation available concering goitrogenic diets as an alternative therapy for Graves' disease (see Chapter 11 for information on diet and dietary iodine).

Anyone with severe TED should discuss with their doctor the use of steroids combined with radioactive iodine therapy or other alternatives. People who cannot take steroids and who have TED should discuss alternative options to radioactive iodine with their doctors, since radioactive iodine can worsen TED.

Informed Consent for Graves' Disease Patients

A common problem for people with Graves' disease is a lack of informed consent—that is, full disclosure of all the treatment options, treatment outcomes, and goals of therapy—prior to therapy. When thyroid patients have severe symptoms, they may not be able to properly take in and appreciate all that is conveyed in a doctor's appointment. Many Graves' patients are shocked to learn that they did not understand what they were told in the doctor's office concerning becoming hypothyroid. And doctors can assume that patients understand when they don't ask questions.

Antithyroid Medication

Sometimes, doctors (or patients) prefer to treat Graves' disease with antithyroid drugs. These drugs prevent the thyroid from manufacturing thyroid hormone and are usually a way of managing Graves' disease in the short term. The two drugs most commonly used are propylthiouracil (PTU) and methimazole (Tapazole). They are very useful to treat specific circumstances, such as:

- Graves' disease in pregnancy
- Severe thyrotoxicosis, to lower the thyroid hormone levels prior to radioactive iodine treatment
- Mild thyrotoxicosis in Graves' disease with a very small goiter
- Severe TED in patients who are reluctant to undergo thyroid surgery
- Thyrotoxicosis in any patient in an unstable clinical condition or in thyroid storm
- Patients who have strong fears about radioactive iodine

Lena's Story: "Why Am I Hypothyroid? I Don't Get It!"

When I was diagnosed with Graves' disease, my doctor recommended radioactive iodine and said that he would give me just enough to make my thyroid normal again and that I wouldn't need medication. After it was all done, I started to feel awful about a month later. I dragged around, was very tired—different than before, when I was exhausted from my hyperthyroidism. I wasn't myself, and I complained to my doctor that the radioactive iodine must have done this. He told me that I had become hypothyroid and would need thyroid hormone medication for the rest of my life. I went in to get rid of my overactive thyroid, and now I had an underactive thyroid!

I was so furious that I went to a lawyer to see if I could sue for malpractice. I saw my lawyer a couple of times, and he said there was no case; he had contacted some expert witnesses and what happened to me is supposed to happen and is "standard of care." I couldn't grasp how this could be, when no one told me this would occur. I went to see three more doctors and now understand that either the first doctor did not correctly explain things to me or else I just didn't have a clue what he was telling me.

As the production of thyroid hormone decreases, the symptoms of thyrotoxicosis will disappear. The practice is to take you off the drugs after several months of treatment if your TSH level is normal or elevated, to see whether Graves' disease relapses or goes into remission. Relapse occurs about 80 percent of the time, but some people like to take their chances at remission. This is a reasonable strategy unless Graves' disease is severe, which for many people can be like a "train wreck."

Remission and Antithyroid Medication

Graves' disease can be easily controlled with antithyroid medication in virtually all patients who are tolerant of these medications. The main benefit of going on antithyroid medication is to try your luck at achieving full remission without the need for radioactive iodine treatment or surgery. This usually results in either an indefinite period of normal thyroid activity or lifelong hypothyroidism thereafter. In general, antithyroid drugs are effective in achieving remission about 20 to 30 percent of the time, but some doctors report lower success rates.

Using antithyroid drugs buys time until either a spontaneous remission occurs or the autoimmune effects destroy enough of the thyroid gland to wear it down despite persistent TSA production. A spontaneous remission (an end to the thyrotoxicosis without taking further medications) is most likely to take place in cases of very mild thyrotoxicosis and small goiters. It takes about six to eight weeks on the medication for the thyroid hormone levels to reach a normal range, and remission occurs by six months to a year, if it is going to happen at all. Although it is possible for remission to take place after longer periods of time, it is better to avoid open-ended treatment courses. Ultimately, there is no advantage to postponing more definitive treatment with radioactive iodine.

Many patients and doctors feel it's worth trying for a full remission initially before more definitive therapies are used. In the end, many of the patients on antithyroid drugs wind up having either radioactive iodine treatment or a thyroidectomy. Signs that antithyroid drugs are failing to provide a remission include:

- TSH levels that remain lower than normal
- Persistently high TSA levels
- A relatively high level of T3 in the blood compared to T4

The Ups and Downs of Antithyroid Medication

There is an upside to antithyroid drugs. Patients with eye problems may experience more improvement in their eyes while on antithyroid medication than with other forms of treatment.

One downside of antithyroid drugs is a small (around 1 percent) risk of destroying the bone marrow (aplastic anemia) or the liver. Another downside is that there is data showing that radioactive iodine therapy doesn't work as well on Graves' disease patients who were treated with the antithyroid medication propylthiouracil (PTU) first. If you're having radioactive iodine therapy after pretreatment with antithyroid medication, the current literature suggests using higher doses of radioactive iodine.

If you have Graves' disease, it's realistic to assume that after treatment you'll need to be put on thyroid hormone replacement for life. The general recommendation is to avoid antithyroid medication if a doctor knows for certain that you'll be having radioactive iodine therapy and your thyrotoxic symptoms are not too severe. Instead, beta-blockers can be used to control some of the symptoms of thyrotoxicosis until the thyroid hormone level is restored to the normal range.

Thyroidectomy or Partial Thyroidectomy

Another treatment for Graves' disease is either a partial or near-total thyroidectomy (surgical removal of the thyroid gland). This is reserved for Graves' patients with a goiter causing obstruction in the neck, for patients for whom there is a concern that a thyroid nodule accompanying Graves' is suspicious for cancer, or for patients who refuse radioactive iodine therapy. A partial or near-total thyroidectomy means that the surgeon deliberately leaves behind remnants of the thyroid gland so that thyroid hormone replacement may not be necessary, although this almost never works. Patients often wind up hypothyroid anyway, since even the remnants of the gland will still burn out from Graves' disease antibodies, if it is severe. If you are considering a partial or near-total thyroidecomy, your physician should make it clear that this will not guarantee "no hypothyroidism," but will rather provide a small chance that hypothyroidism will not occur.

In a total thyroidectomy, essentially the entire gland is removed. There are generally more risks involved with thyroidectomy than with radioactive iodine therapy for Graves' disease, which is why this is not the first line therapy for most Graves' patients. It is important to keep in mind that the risks of surgery (discussed in Chapter 6) are *higher* than any perceived risks of radioactive iodine therapy.

Spontaneous Remission of Graves' Disease

There are rare cases in which Graves' disease can go into remission without any treatment, which may explain why some people go into

Be Informed: Hypothyroidism Following Graves' Disease Treatment

Many Graves' patients are outraged or just surprised to find out that they are hypothyroid after radioactive iodine therapy for Graves' disease. In fact, hypothyroidism is the end goal and *raison d'être* of this therapy for Graves' disease. Radioactive iodine therapy treats hyperthyroidism caused by Graves' disease by destroying (ablating) the thyroid gland, which causes it to stop producing thyroid hormone. No one should be advised that the thyroid gland will be "normal" after this therapy, although in rare cases hypothyroidism does not immediately occur and normal thyroid function may resume without thyroid hormone replacement therapy at first.

Before consenting to radioactive treatment, be sure to discuss the outcome with your doctor until you have all the information you need and understand what will result from the therapy. If you're hypothyroid after radioactive therapy, that's good news. The therapy worked, and you will no longer suffer from the harmful effects of hyperthyroidism and thyrotoxicosis. At this point, being placed on the proper dose of levothyroxine will restore you to normal. For more information on radioactive iodine, see Chapter 9.

remission on antithyroid medication. This has led many people to think that remission can always occur, which is not the case. If a person's thyrotoxicosis is mild enough to be controlled on beta-blockers alone, the rate of remission is similar to people on antithyroid drugs over the same period of time.

It's been theorized that removing certain stressors, which may have triggered the autoimmune disease in the first place, could help lead to spontaneous remission. This is unproven, but it is useful to review some of the stress reduction techniques described in Chapter 12, which covers complementary medicine.

Euthyroid Graves' Disease

Euthyroid Graves' disease involves cases in which there are no symptoms of thyrotoxicosis in spite of Graves' disease. In these instances, patients are noted to have the bulging eyes of Graves' ophthalmopathy, but their thyroid glands are still working normally. Many of these people will ultimately develop thyrotoxicosis; however, some never do. In this situation, the approach calls for watching and waiting. Physicians will watch patients' eyes for changes (see Chapter 7) and routinely monitor thyroid hormone levels to prevent thyrotoxicosis.

Allowing Graves' Disease to Run Its Natural Course

There are many people with Graves' disease who have mild symptoms and who wonder whether they should refuse active therapy and allow Graves' disease to run its natural course. This approach would likely result in the thyroid gland burning itself out and failing on its own, resulting in hypothyroidism anyway. This approach is commonly recommended for the small group of people who have such low degrees of thyrotoxicosis that ablative therapy with radioactive iodine, surgery, or the risks of side effects of antithyroid medications seem unnecessary. These people often do well with beta-blockers; however, they must be carefully monitored since thyrotoxicosis may worsen without warning.

Other Causes of Thyrotoxicosis

There are other causes of thyrotoxicosis besides hyperthyroidism. This section covers the three most common: autonomous toxic nodules (ATNs), toxic multinodular goiter, and thyroid hormone overdose.

Autonomous Toxic Nodules

Autonomous toxic nodules (ATNs), also known as toxic adenomas, or autonomous toxic thyroid nodules, are single thyroid nodules that independently make too much thyroid hormone without the need for TSH to stimulate them. These ATNs are suspected when people are thyrotoxic, their TSH level is low, and their thyroid gland has a lump or nodule. A radioactive iodine thyroid scan is used to diagnose a toxic nodule. (See Chapter 5.)

Toxic Multinodular Goiter

Some people's thyroid glands form multiple nodules, which can usually be felt via a physical examination of their thyroid. For much the same reason as in singular toxic adenomas, these multiple thyroid nodules produce too much thyroid hormone and do not require TSH to do so. In such a situation, the radioactive iodine thyroid scan will show multiple toxic thyroid nodules, termed a *toxic multinodular goiter.*

Thyroid Hormone Overdose

Thyroid hormone overdose is a common problem. One reason is because dosages of thyroid hormone used for treatment may not be based on appropriate monitoring using appropriate laboratory tests. This results in some people remaining hypothyroid with inadequate thyroid hormone dosages, while others become thyrotoxic with too much thyroid hormone.

Poor compliance is the second most common reason for overdose. Sometimes thyroid patients experience memory loss problems; they may forget that they have taken their thyroid hormone pill and repeat the dosage. Other people mistakenly believe that purposely taking excessive thyroid hormone doses will alleviate symptoms of tiredness and lack of energy. Ironically, these symptoms are worsened by this deliberate overdose.

People treated for thyroid cancer need to be on higher doses of thyroid hormone to suppress TSH. Sometimes, if poorly adjusted, these higher doses can result in thyrotoxicosis. Thyroid cancer and TSH suppression dosing is discussed more in Chapter 10.

Misuse of Thyroid Hormone

Thyroid hormone has a shady history of inappropriate uses in the past. Throughout the 1950s, 1960s, and even 1970s, overweight or obese women were frequently prescribed levothyroxine sodium as a weight-loss drug and told that it would speed up their metabolisms, resulting in the desired weight loss. This practice is known as off-label prescribing and was the source of countless cases of thyrotoxicosis, which frequently went untreated, imperiling these women. Some weight-loss supplements, which are not regulated by the FDA, contain mostly active thyroid hormone; you should be especially suspect about diet supplements that claim that you can "eat all you want and still lose weight."

Thyroiditis

As mentioned previously, thyroiditis means "inflammation of the thyroid gland." Some types of thyroiditis can cause thyrotoxicosis. This is discussed further in Chapter 4.

Hamburger Toxicosis

There have been rare cases in which ingesting ground meat, such as hamburger, containing thyroid tissue has caused isolated outbreaks of thyrotoxicosis. In one incident in the mid-1980s, for example, some members of an entire community suddenly developed thyrotoxicosis. Upon investigation, the outbreak was linked to a meat packing plant that had made hamburger from the neck muscles of cattle, thus contaminating it with thyroid tissue.

Diagnosing Thyrotoxicosis and/or Hyperthyroidism

Thyrotoxicosis can be easily diagnosed when there is elevated free T4 or T3 levels and a TSH level that is lower than normal (usually less than 0.2). See Chapter 2 for more details on lab testing for TSH and free T4 and T3.

The challenge for diagnosing either hyperthyroidism and/or thyrotoxicosis is similar for hypothyroidism: the symptoms can overlap with stress, anxiety, panic disorder, low blood sugar, and cardiovascular diseases. For women, PMS and perimenopause can mask or be mistaken for thyrotoxicosis; miscarriage or infertility can also result from thyrotoxicosis.

A Word About Panic Attacks

Some people experience a panic attack as "choking" symptoms: rapid breathing or hyperventilating; a perception of difficult breathing, choking, a smothering sensation, or a lump in the throat; and chest pain, pressure, or discomfort. Roughly 2 percent of North Americans ages eighteen to fifty-four suffer from panic attacks each year, and they occur twice as often in women as they do in men. It is not known, however, how many of the people who suffer from panic disorder are thyrotoxic. If you begin to suffer from panic attacks, make sure to have your thyroid levels checked to rule out thyrotoxicosis as an underlying cause.

Testing for Antibodies

If you are not hypothyroid and thyrotoxicosis from too much medication is not an issue, then it's important to find out whether you have autoimmune thyroid disease. You may have the beginnings of Hashimoto's disease (and Hashitoxicosis, discussed in Chapter 2), or you may have Graves' disease. Testing for thyroid autoantibodies (see pages 43–45) will help to determine whether you have autoimmune thyroid disease, which could be causing thyrotoxicosis. This involves a simple blood test.

Treating Thyrotoxicosis Not Caused by Graves' Disease

Treating thyrotoxicosis may be simple or very complex, depending on the cause. If the cause of your thyrotoxicosis is too high a dosage of thyroid hormone medication, then the dosage is lowered. In addition, you may be placed on a beta-blocker to stop the adrenaline rush symptoms that are responsible for a racing heart, panic, and so on. It would be critical to have your thyroid hormone dose readjusted to make sure that the TSH is normal when checked at least eight weeks later. If you are taking T3 in addition to T4, then you should probably stop taking T3 and your TSH levels should be rechecked.

If the cause of thyrotoxicosis is hyperthyroidism, then the exact cause has to be found to determine treatment options. You may be placed on a beta-blocker and antithyroid medication until you can be treated with radioactive iodine or surgery. In some instances of thyroiditis, the thyrotoxicosis resolves on its own and runs its course; if this is the case, you may just need to "hang out" on a beta-blocker.

More About Beta-Blockers

Thyrotoxicosis increases the body's sensitivity to adrenaline by increasing the number of beta-adrenergic receptors (beta receptors) in many of the cells of the body. This results in many of the symptoms associated with thyrotoxicosis, particularly rapid heart rate, palpitations, and anxiety. Blocking these beta receptors can alleviate these symptoms and prevent severe effects on the heart. Beta-blockers are drugs that block the effect of the body's own adrenaline on activating these receptors. They include propranolol, metoprolol, atenolol, and many others, all of which are in the -*olol* family of medications. Beta receptors come in two types. Beta-1 receptors increase the heart rate, while beta-2 receptors open up airways. If you are asthmatic or have emphysema, you may need special beta-blockers that only block the beta-1 receptor, because blockage of beta-2 receptors would make you severely short of breath. If you have severe asthma, you may not be able to tolerate any type of beta-blocker.

Although beta-blockers are usually very well tolerated, there are rare side effects, such as rashes or other reactions. The most disturbing side effect is reversible hair loss (alopecia). Very rarely, hair can begin to fall out several months after beginning to take a beta-blocker; the hair follicles are intact, but somehow the hair cycle is disturbed, going into a continuous shedding process. If this occurs, the hair will grow back when you go off the beta-blocker, but it may take a long time or not grow back as full as it was. Many doctors are unaware of this side effect and may tell you that your hair is thinning for other reasons. In general, thyroid-related hair loss is usually attributed to hypothyroidism or hyperthyroidism, but a small number of women may experience it from a beta-blocker.

Valeria's Story: Hair Loss on My Beta-Blocker

I am a thyroid cancer survivor and am on a TSH-suppression dose of levothyroxine, because my TSH needs to be zero. I started to have all the thyrotoxic symptoms, including a sort of low blood sugar feeling; if I didn't eat regularly, I would start to get shaky and irritable, and my pulse was always about 100. My doctor put me on a beta-blocker, which took my pulse from 100 down to 70. I felt much better and I was able to go a longer time without eating! After being on the drug for about nine months, I started to notice that my hair was falling out. I would grasp my ponytail and *clumps* of hair would come out. It was everywhere—on my pillow at night, in the shower, and when I combed my hair. It started to be very noticeable, and I had to get a wig. I was told that it was just "aging" and probably due to menopause.

Since the beta-blocker was the only new medication I had started, I looked it up in the *Physician's Desk Reference*; sure enough, under "rare side effects," I saw "reversible alopecia." I was weaned off the drug, and about three months later, all this new stubble started to grow in. My doctor said he had never seen this before, but when he surveyed other patients on beta-blockers, a few of them said their hair was falling out, too. Since hair loss is caused by so many things, this cause apparently gets missed.

4

Thyroiditis

Inflammation of the Thyroid Gland

IN THE UNITED States alone, roughly forty million people are affected by thyroiditis. Just as *tonsillitis* refers to inflamed tonsils, *thyroiditis* refers to an inflamed thyroid gland. Depending on what kind of thyroiditis you have, a goiter and symptoms of thyrotoxicosis or hypothyroidism can develop. The most common type of thyroiditis is Hashimoto's thyroiditis, an autoimmune disorder discussed in Chapter 2, which affects roughly one in five women. This chapter explains other kinds of thyroid inflammation in more detail and discusses the forms thyroiditis can take.

The best way to understand thyroiditis is to think of it in terms of a swollen gland. In the same way that the lymph nodes or salivary glands swell because of various viral infections, the thyroid, too, can swell. In fact, after Hashimoto's disease, the main cause of thyroiditis is viral infection. In very rare cases, bacterial infections may require hospitalization and intravenous antibiotic therapy.

Subacute Viral Thyroiditis: Pain in the Neck!

Subacute viral thyroiditis is also known as *de Quervain's thyroiditis*, after the Swiss physician who first described it. This form of thyroiditis seems to be particularly prevalent in North America, although

Hashimoto's disease is about forty times more common. It is more common in women than in men. Subacute (or "not-so-severe") viral thyroiditis is probably caused by one or more viruses. Although there is no final proof that this condition is viral in origin, several possible viruses that are similar to the measles or mumps viruses and to certain common cold viruses have been implicated.

De Quervain's thyroiditis ranges from extremely mild to severe and runs its course the way a normal flu virus does. If you have a mild case of viral thyroiditis, you will probably not even bother to see a doctor, because he or she won't notice any symptoms other than perhaps a sore throat. In more severe cases, however, you can be extremely uncomfortable.

Subacute viral thyroiditis usually imitates the flu; you'll be tired and have muscular aches and pains, a headache, and a fever. As the illness progresses, however, your thyroid gland will swell or enlarge from the infection and become very tender. It will hurt to swallow, and you might feel stabs of pain in your neck. To make matters worse, you can also become thyrotoxic. When the gland gets inflamed, thyroid hormones leak out of the thyroid gland the way pus oozes out of a blister in a similar way to what happens with Hashitoxicosis (see Chapter 2). Your system will have too much thyroid hormone in it, and you will experience all the classic thyrotoxicosis symptoms outlined in Chapter 3.

On the positive side, subacute thyroiditis is temporary and even the more severe cases tend to run their course in about six weeks. It can be a miserable six weeks, however, particularly if you don't know what's wrong. Although the condition can take longer to clear up, it's very unusual for it to linger beyond six months.

If you go to your doctors with the complaint of a sore throat, the diagnosis may be missed unless you point out exactly where the swelling and tenderness is coming from. Often, though, the thyrotoxicosis symptoms of viral thyroiditis are what would bring you to the doctor.

Subacute viral thyroiditis is diagnosed in part through the process of elimination, after ruling out Graves' disease and Hashimoto's thyroiditis. Because your thyroid gland is tender, the doctor should know it isn't Graves' disease. Hashimoto's thyroiditis is often suspected;

however, it is not associated with a tender, painful thyroid gland. A blood test can easily rule out Hashimoto's disease because there would be no antibodies present in your blood. Your thyroid hormone levels and thyroglobulin (Tg) levels would be very high because of the hormones leaking out of the inflamed thyroid gland.

In more severe instances, where a goiter may be present, radioactive iodine uptake tests are performed (see Chapter 9). A normal range for the uptake is 8 to 30 percent absorption; with viral thyroiditis, the uptake is less than1 percent because the infected thyroid cells are too sick to absorb the iodine. But since the condition runs its course, uptake tests are probably excessive. Nonspecific tests of inflammation in the body—the erythrocyte sedimentation rate (ESR) and the C-reactive protein (CRP)—are usually both quite high with this condition. Sometimes, particularly if the thyroid gland is irregular and needs to be checked for a possible cancer, a fine needle aspiration biopsy can diagnose de Quervain's thyroiditis.

For mild cases of viral thyroiditis, the treatment is aspirin to alleviate the swelling and inflammation. If the thyrotoxicosis is more severe, a beta-blocker may be given to slow your heart rate. In more severe forms, cortisone analogs are given, such as prednisone. Sometimes the inflammation causes temporary damage to the thyroid cells and hypothyroidism can set in. If this happens, a temporary dosage of thyroid hormone is prescribed until the hypothyroidism corrects itself. Generally, as the infection inflammation clears up, the thyroid gland resumes its normal, healthy function; only 10 percent of de Quervain's thyroiditis cases result in permanent hypothyroidism.

Silent Thyroiditis

The silent form of thyroiditis is so named because it's tricky to diagnose and often avoids detection until symptoms become severe. It is debatable whether this is a unique type of thyroiditis or a type of Hashimoto's thyroiditis that is not associated with a goiter. Since most forms of autoimmune thyroiditis that present with lymphocytes invading the thyroid gland (lymphocytic thyroiditis) are commonly called Hashimoto's thyroiditis, the differences between these two labels might be insignificant. Silent thyroiditis runs a painless course but is otherwise similar to subacute viral thyroiditis and essentially the same as Hashitoxicosis. With this version, there are no symptoms or outward signs of inflammation, but mild thyrotoxicosis still occurs for the same hormone leakage.

There is no evidence that a virus is involved in silent thyroiditis. There are some who think this type of thyroiditis might be a short-lived autoimmune disorder, like a mini-Hashimoto's disease. Silent thyroiditis sufferers are usually women, and it commonly occurs post-partum. (Postpartum thyroiditis, discussed in the upcoming section and in Chapter 8, is silent thyroiditis after delivery.)

In the course of the diagnosis, a silent thyroiditis sufferer may be given a radioactive iodine uptake test. The uptake test can reveal the real cause of the hyperthyroidism, showing very low absorption.

As with de Quervain's thyroiditis, silent thyroiditis usually runs its course and the thyrotoxicosis clears up. Beta-blockers may provide relief from some thyrotoxic symptoms. If a period of hypothyroidism follows the transient episode of thyrotoxicosis, thyroid hormone treatment may be required unless the episode was very brief. Some people with silent thyroiditis become permanently hypothyroid, requiring lifelong thyroid hormone replacement therapy.

Postpartum Thyroiditis

Postpartum thyroiditis is a general label referring to silent thyroiditis after delivery, which causes mild hyperthyroidism, and a short-lived Hashimoto's-type of thyroiditis that causes mild hypothyroidism. Women with thyroid peroxidase (TPO) antibodies are more likely to experience postpartum thyroiditis. Until quite recently, the mild hypothyroid and mild thyrotoxicosis symptoms were simply attributed to the symptoms of postpartum depression—the notorious post-partum blues—thought to be caused by the dramatic hormonal and emotional changes women experience after pregnancy. But recent studies indicate that just under 20 percent of all pregnant women experience transient thyroid problems and subsequent mild forms of thyrotoxicosis or hypothyroidism. See Chapter 8 for more information on postpartum thyroiditis.

Maya's Story: "It's Normal to Feel Tired"

After I had my little boy, I found that I was losing my baby weight without difficulty, but then I started to notice that my heart was racing and I had a sort of exhausted feeling all the time. I was told that this was normal. Then I started to feel really fatigued and sort of foggy and down, and I noticed that I was becoming constipated. At my three-month appointment with my doctor, she told me that I had all the classic signs of postpartum blues and that "it's normal to feel tired" after having a baby. I started to feel better in about a month. Then, at my next routine exam, my doctor noticed that my thyroid was enlarged and checked into it. I had normal TSH, but they found TPO antibodies, even though I was feeling fine. My doctor explained that I probably had a "minithyroid problem" that went away on its own. She said that it was probably enlarged earlier, but she probably missed it. She explained that this type of thyroid condition is so short lived, the only treatment would have been just for symptom relief—beta-blockers for my hyperthyroidism and then some thyroid hormone for the hypothyroidism.

Acute Suppurative Thyroiditis

Also known simply as acute bacterial thyroiditis, acute supperative thyroiditis is a very rare condition—so rare that even thyroid specialists may never see a single case in their career. When it does occur, it's usually seen in children.

The term *suppurative* refers to the presence of bacteria and pus; in this condition, the thyroid gland suffers a dramatic pus-forming bacterial infection similar to the ones that cause boils and abscesses. The thyroid gland becomes painful and inflamed, and a high fever and chills accompany the infection. Sometimes an abscess within the gland contains pus. The tenderness of the thyroid gland is usually obvious, so it's difficult to miss the symptoms. A fine needle biopsy can provide abscess material to examine for bacteria. Antibiotics, incision, and drainage are the treatments.

Riedel's Thyroiditis

Riedel's thyroiditis is the rarest form of thyroiditis. In this condition the thyroid gland is infiltrated by scar tissue throughout the gland, which binds it to surrounding portions of the neck. The thyroid will feel tender and become very hard like wood. Hence, the terms *ligneous* (woody) or *fibrous* (scar tissue) thyroiditis are also used to describe this peculiar condition. Because the gland attaches itself to overlying skin and deeper structures in the neck, your windpipe might feel constricted and your vocal cords could be affected as well. Your voice might become husky and swallowing could become difficult.

The diagnosis for this disorder usually involves a biopsy to rule out cancer, but the cause of the condition itself is unknown. The only treatment option is surgical removal of the front part of the gland itself. Since this condition is so rare, the portions of the thyroid that are removed during surgery must be evaluated by specialist pathologists with expertise in thyroid pathology.

5

Thyroid Nodules

Lumps in the Thyroid Gland

IN THE CONTEXT of thyroid disease, the word *nodule* means "lump in the thyroid gland." If a lump is in your neck but outside your thyroid gland, it is just a lump and not a nodule, and usually refers to an enlarged lymph node.

Most thyroid cancers are first found as nodules in the thyroid gland or as lumps or enlarged lymph nodes in other places in the neck. Getting a lump checked out gives you the opportunity to discover and treat a thyroid cancer early, should it turn out to be cancer. But since most thyroid nodules are benign, getting it checked may allow you to quickly put your fears of cancer to rest.

Some benign thyroid nodules, called autonomous toxic nodules (ATN), make thyroid hormone in greater than normal amounts, without being controlled by the pituitary gland through its thyroid-stimulating hormone secretion. If there are multiple ATNs in your gland, it's called a toxic multinodular goiter. Most thyroid nodules are colloid nodules, which are benign. Colloid nodules do not produce too much thyroid hormone and usually do not require treatment once they are identified.

Sometimes a thyroid nodule is shown to be a bag of fluid within the gland called a *cyst*. Other times the nodule is a complex cyst, which means that it is partly cystic and partly solid. Most cysts are benign, but some contain thyroid cancer in the wall of the cyst. Likewise, complex cysts are usually benign but sometimes contain thyroid cancers.

This chapter will walk you through the process of discovering and evaluating a thyroid nodule. Not everyone who is diagnosed with thyroid cancer will go through a thyroid nodule investigation because cancer may be discovered only after it has spread to different sites in the body. However, those who do have nodules investigated will have the opportunity to find thyroid cancers at an early stage.

Finding a Thyroid Nodule

Single thyroid nodules are usually one of three things: a cyst, which is a growth that contains fluid; a benign tumor or adenoma, which is a growth that contains abnormal, noncancerous cells; or a carcinoma, which is a growth that contains abnormal, cancerous cells. As already mentioned, cysts are frequently benign, and the majority of thyroid nodules are also benign.

Most thyroid nodules are discovered as obvious nodules in the lower front of the neck, seen by the person or by a friend or family member. A physician may also find a nodule during a physical examination. A complaint of a sore throat, for example, usually completely unrelated to the nodule, may prompt such an exam, resulting in the nodule being found by accident. In addition, if you were exposed to radiation therapy to your neck during childhood, you are at risk for developing thyroid cancer. In this case, you should have regular thyroid exams to detect thyroid nodules that could be cancerous. You can also do your own thyroid self-exam, which is discussed later in the chapter.

When investigating a thyroid nodule, size matters! For that reason, a nodule with the size of 1.0 cm (0.4 in.) in diameter or less is considered too small to be significant and usually does not need further evaluation.

Thyroid Self-Exam

Every year, thousands of women find breast cancer nodules by doing breast self-exams. The thyroid self-exam (TSE) follows the same idea and is also known as the "neck check." All you'll need is a glass of water and a hand-held mirror. Here are the standard steps:

1. Hold the mirror in your hand, focusing on the area of your neck just below the Adam's apple. The Adam's Apple (which some people confuse with the thyroid gland) is the thyroid cartiledge. Both men and women have it, but it is larger and more prominent in a man. It is found immediately above the collarbone.
2. While focusing on this area in the mirror, tip your head back slightly.
3. Take a drink of water and swallow. Normally, as you swallow, your windpipe raises and then goes back to its normal position.
4. As you swallow, look at your neck. Check for any bulges or a protrusion in this area when you swallow. (The thyroid gland is located further down on your neck, closer to the collarbone.) Repeat this a few times to be sure you're all clear.

Over and Above the Standard TSE

- Place your fingers at the back of your neck, at the top of your spine, and then knead your neck tissue toward the front like a piece of raw dough, feeling all the way around to the front of your throat. Work the right side of your neck from back to front center and then the left side from back to front center. You're searching for a painless nodule anywhere from the size of a pea to the size of a golf ball.
- Feel all around the area just above your collarbone, or "pocket." Again, you're looking for a painless nodule.

If you notice any bulges or nodules in these areas, see your doctor as soon as possible to have your nodule investigated. In addition, if you have swollen lymph nodes in your neck or under your ears that persist for longer than one month, you need to get them evaluated by a doctor. Your doctor can tell you whether the nodule is in the thyroid.

Evaluating a Nodule

There are three crucial tests to properly evaluate a thyroid nodule. The first is a TSH test, and the second is an ultrasound imaging test to determine the size of the nodule. The third is a fine needle aspiration (FNA), which draws cells and fluids from the nodule for evaluation by a pathologist.

The TSH Test: Why You Need One

The TSH test (see Chapter 2) will immediately tell you whether your nodule is an autonomous toxic nodule (ATN). It *cannot* be an ATN if your TSH level is not suppressed (under 0.2). Furthermore, if your TSH level is suppressed, it can save you from having to have an FNA; the only type of nodule that can be treated without the need for a biopsy is an ATN because it is very unlikely to be cancer. Any other thyroid nodule that is larger than 1.0 cm (0.4 in.) in diameter requires an FNA biopsy.

Thus, the diagnostic course is set by the TSH test. If the TSH is low (less than 0.2), then the next step is a radioactive iodine thyroid scan (see Chapter 9). This scan will show whether the nodule you've discovered is hot, meaning that it sucks up most of the radioactive iodine. If it is a hot nodule, then a biopsy is not needed and you can be reasonably confident that this is an ATN. If the rest of the thyroid is hot but the nodule is *not* hot, then the nodule should be biopsied. This situation could be seen if a person has Graves' disease as well as a thyroid nodule. In this case, the nodule could be benign (colloid nodule or cyst), or it could be a thyroid cancer, although this would be rare. If it were malignant, then surgical removal of the entire gland would be appropriate for both the Graves' disease and the cancer. The best test to ascertain the nature of the nodule in this situation is a fine needle aspiration biopsy

Ultrasound: Sizing up the Situation

An ultrasound is a device that uses high-frequency sound waves to produce an echo picture of structures in your body. It is the same type

Su Lin's Story: A Pediatric Blunder

I like to think I'm an attentive parent, and when my ten-year-old daughter showed me a lump on the side of her neck, I brought this to the attention of her pediatrician. He prescribed antibiotics, which did not seem to change the lump. Six months later, my daughter started to complain about a "weird feeling" when she swallowed her food. So I took my daughter back to the pediatrician, and he felt the lump and told us it was a nodule on her thyroid gland. He gave us more antibiotics and told us to come back in four weeks to see if the nodule had shrunk. Nothing changed. The pediatrician sent my daughter for a thyroid scan, and the thyroid scan was apparently normal.

I was getting really frustrated, because the lump just wouldn't go away and was getting bigger. We were finally referred to a surgeon, who removed the nodule, and then we learned it was thyroid cancer. My daughter was immediately booked for a thyroidectomy and lymph node resection. She walked around with this cancer for almost a year and a half because her pediatrician didn't diagnose her properly! If I could do it all over again, I'd insist on better care: a TSH test and an FNA could have saved us dangerously wasted time.

of machine used to look at a fetus within a mother's womb. A jelly lubricant is smeared on the neck to allow the ultrasound transducer to slide easily over your skin. The picture produced by the ultrasound machine produces an excellent image of the thyroid gland so that any nodules or masses can be assessed and measured. A fine needle biopsy can be performed during the ultrasound to obtain samples of cells from the nodule or mass, permitting the physician to find out whether it is malignant.

Although most thyroid nodules can be biopsied by a skilled physician without an ultrasound, sometimes thyroid nodules are discovered accidentally while performing an ultrasound evaluation of the carotid arteries and the nodule can only be found with the ultrasound. A major problem with thyroid ultrasound evaluations is that these devices are much too sensitive. Most people can be shown to have very tiny thyroid nodules using a thyroid ultrasound. When a physical examination is used to find thyroid nodules to evaluate for possible cancer, only large and clinically significant nodules (usually greater than 1.0 cm in diameter) can be found. These types of nodules have a 10 percent chance of being malignant and so warrant a biopsy.

Should Ultrasounds Be Used to Screen for Thyroid Nodules?

Very tiny nodules are found in nearly all people during ultrasound exams. Since these tiny nodules have such a small chance of being anything to worry about, it's just not feasible to check them out in everybody. For this reason, thyroid ultrasounds should not be used to screen for thyroid nodules in most people because you'll almost always find them. The only population that warrants screening is the population that has been exposed to radiation in the neck or exposed to fallout from nuclear testing. People with a history of childhood exposure to radiation therapy in the neck region or to radiation fallout from nuclear testing are three times more likely to develop thyroid cancer than those in the general population, so finding nodules in these people could help to find early thyroid cancers (see "Who Should be Screened for Thyroid Nodules" in this chapter).

Fine Needle Aspiration Biopsy: The Gold Standard

Fine needle aspiration has changed the way thyroid nodules are biopsied and evaluated. Thirty years ago, thyroid nodules were usually tested with a radioactive iodine scan without a TSH test to see if the nodule was hot or cold. Painful core biopsies, using a thick needle, were also used.

FNA has changed all that. FNA, a twenty-minute procedure, is usually very accurate. It can be performed in a doctor's office and is as simple as drawing a blood sample. It is considered the gold standard for evaluating a thyroid nodule. Studies have shown that because of FNA, cases of thyroid surgery have dropped by 50 percent. This means that many people can be spared "look-see" surgery, which used to be done frequently when cancer was suspected.

Before an FNA, the skin around your nodule is cleansed with antiseptic. The needle, which is thinner than the standard needles used to sample blood, needs to be inserted three to six times to obtain a good sample. This is known as obtaining passes and means that each nodule is aspirated in different areas and in different directions. If you have several nodules, they'll each need to be aspirated with the appropriate number of passes, and greater attention will be paid to larger nodules. The needle will aspirate, or draw out, cells and/or fluid, which are sent off to a pathologist to determine whether the nodule is benign or malignant.

Once the aspiration is done, you'll get a bandage on the puncture site and then go home. You may have some neck tenderness or mild swelling afterward, but that will subside within twenty-four hours. If you develop a fever or notice the puncture site is black and blue or bleeding, call your doctor. This may mean that you have a broken blood vessel or an infection at the puncture site.

FNA Accuracy

Like many diagnostic procedures used to detect cancer, including Pap smears and mammograms, FNA is not 100 percent accurate. Any physician, including endocrinologists, internists, surgeons, pathologists, and radiologists, can perform FNAs if they're trained in the procedure. But fine needle aspiration is not an exact science. Much depends on the skill of the doctor performing the FNA, his or her ability to obtain an adequate specimen of the right area, and the experience of the pathologist reading the slide that contains the smear. As a result, there are often inconclusive or unsatisfactory results.

A result that's inconclusive means that there's no way for the pathologist to tell whether the nodule is benign or malignant. This happens about 10 to 15 percent of the time. In these cases, the slides are sometimes sent to a pathologist or cytologist who has more experience in interpreting cells. He or she can review the slides as well as interpret them. The other options in these cases are either to wait and repeat the FNA or to go directly to surgery, depending upon the size and characteristics of the nodule. An unsatisfactory result, which happens 1 to 10 percent of the time, means that the FNA procedure was not successful in obtaining enough thyroid cells for the pathologist to make a diagnosis. In this case, the FNA may need to be repeated.

Other common pathology errors include:

- Calling tissue malignant when it's benign. This is called a false positive.
- Calling tissue benign when it's malignant. This is called a false negative.
- Identifying the malignant tumor correctly, but not classifying it as the right cell type or grade.
- Calling inadequate FNA samples benign because no cancer cells are seen. To be considered benign, the slides must contain sufficient numbers of noncancerous thyroid cells.

Since pathology errors are common, a second opinion is advised when cancer is in question.

Confirming a Pathology Report

The only way to confirm a cancer diagnosis is through a biopsy of the tissue. If you receive news that your nodule is (or might be) cancerous, make sure to get a second pathologist with equal or more experience to review the biopsy slides and provide an independent, separate opinion.

Types of Thyroid Nodules

The good news is that 90 percent of all thyroid nodules turn out to be benign. Nodules are often benign if you discover more than one of them or if the rest of the thyroid gland itself is enlarged. Benign nodules also tend to be fleshier and softer, like the tip of your nose, while cancerous nodules tend to be hard, like the tip of your elbow. There are many kinds of benign nodules that could be caused by thyroiditis (see Chapters 2 and 4), while normal thyroid gland tissue could also cause a benign colloid nodule.

Benign Thyroid Nodules

The most common type of benign thyroid nodule is a colloid nodule, which is made up of normal thyroid tissue. Again, the size of the nodule matters, and it should be measured because a colloid nodule will often shrink. If the nodule is positioned in a way that makes it difficult to measure, an ultrasound can be used to document its size.

A nodule should be reevaluated after eight to ten months to see if it has grown larger. If the nodule shrinks, then the diagnosis of benign colloid nodule is confirmed. This type of nodule needs no further evaluation or concern. However, a large thyroid nodule (over 3.0 cm) that stays the same size over eight to ten months or a nodule of any size that grows larger needs to be biopsied again.

Sometimes, despite several benign biopsies, continuous enlargement of a nodule necessitates thyroid surgery. This is due to two potential problems. First, the nodule could push on vital structures in the neck, such as the windpipe, esophagus, and arteries, causing thoracic outlet obstruction. Second, the continued growth of the nodule could suggest the presence of thyroid cancer despite the results of the biopsy. Because of this, the surgeon should remove at least the half of the thyroid gland involved in the nodule, permitting the pathologist to make a definitive diagnosis.

Thyroid Cysts

As with nodules, size matters for thyroid cysts, and there is no need to worry about small cysts of 1.0 cm (0.4 in.) or less in diameter. When a cyst is larger than this, you'll need to have it evaluated properly for two reasons. First, it might contain a thyroid cancer growing from the wall of the cyst or from the solid portion of a complex nodule. Second, the cyst might grow quite large and cause pain or discomfort, as cysts can sometimes enlarge rapidly. For this reason, the FNA biopsy is performed *after* placing a thin needle into the cyst and sucking out the cyst fluid with a syringe. The cyst fluid might be a straw-colored, chocolate brown, or greenish liquid. It can be watery and thin or thick with blood. Once the cyst is completely drained, a FNA biopsy is performed on the cyst's walls or solid components.

After the cyst is drained of fluid, it might seem to disappear completely. Sometimes the fluid gradually reaccumulates at times making the cyst even larger than before. If this happens, a procedure called cyst sclerosis might be performed. This is a technique in which a mildly irritating liquid is injected into the cyst to make the inside of the cyst walls sticky so that they adhere to each other, eliminating the cyst space. Alternatively, a surgeon may perform a thyroid lobectomy, in which the half of the gland with the cyst is removed, although this is usually done if there is a complex cyst that contains a relatively large solid portion.

Adenomas

An adenoma is a clump of thyroid cells that mass together in a harmless, benign nodule. Since the FNA biopsy appearance of follicular adenomas is similar to that of follicular cancers, most of these nodules require thyroid surgery to be properly classified.

Autonomous Toxic Nodules

As discussed earlier in this chapter, an autonomous toxic nodule (ATN) acts like an independent thyroid gland, making its own thyroid hormone without being controlled by the pituitary gland. Defective TSH receptors get stuck in the on position, so the hormone "switch" is never turned off. The nodule is toxic (not to be confused with malignant) in this case because it causes thyrotoxicosis, making too much thyroid hormone.

Checking the TSH level is the first step in diagnosing an ATN. Most of these nodules do not get biopsied because they show up as hot nodules on radioactive iodine scans (see Chapter 9). Sometimes there are few or no symptoms of thyrotoxicosis and the nodule is very tiny. In this situation, beta-blockers (see Chapter 3) can buy you some time before you get definitive treatment. Otherwise, there are two appropriate choices of definitive therapy: radioactive iodine or thyroid surgery. It is not a good idea to use antithyroid drugs in this situation because these nodules will continue to grow and do not have remissions as can occur with Graves' disease.

Be Informed: The Myth
of the Benign Multinodular Goiter

Some endocrinologists and other primary care doctors seem
to assume that a multinodular goiter, by definition, means
that the largest, or dominant, nodules are benign. This is *not*
true. There may be some nodules that are benign and some
that are malignant.

If you are told you have a multinodular goiter, make
sure to request that the nodules be biopsied. Several patients
with multinodular goiters have been given thyroid hormone
to shrink the goiter when in fact their nodules were cancerous. For example, a fifty-two-year old woman was told she
had a multinodular goiter and put on thyroid hormone for
six years, while the nodule grew larger. Eventually, she consulted another doctor for a second opinion, and that biopsy
revealed thyroid cancer.

Radioactive iodine (RAI) treatment, discussed in Chapter 9, can
be used to treat ATNs. If the ATN is very large, 5.0 cm (2.0 in.) or
more in diameter; if you are pregnant; if radioactive iodine treatment
has not worked well; or if you are reluctant to use radioactive iodine,
then the ATN can be surgically removed. In these cases, it is preferable to remove the entire thyroid lobe rather than just the part of the
lobe containing the ATN. After treatment, thyrotoxicosis clears up
quickly, usually within a week or two. There may be a brief period of
hypothyroidism (see Chapter 2) as the pituitary gland "wakes up" to
make thyroid-stimulating hormone and the remaining thyroid gland
responds to the TSH.

Multinodular Goiters: Toxic and Nontoxic

As discussed earlier, when there are several ATNs on the thyroid
gland, it's called a toxic multinodular goiter. A toxic multinodular
goiter causes hyperthyroidism and all the symptoms of thyrotoxicosis.
Toxic multinodular goiters are usually benign, and, on a radioactive

scan, the multiple nodules will be hot. In these cases, the thyroid gland is treated with either radioactive iodine or surgery.

There are also multinodular goiters made up of non-toxic nodules. It does not cause hyperthyroidism. With a multinodular goiter, each individual nodule must be evaluated, as they are *not* always benign. In these cases, FNA should be performed.

Malignant Thyroid Nodules

About 10 percent of the time, a nodule will be diagnosed as an adenocarcinoma. *Carcinoma* refers to a malignant growth that involves the epithelial cells. But when a tumor in a glandular area is malignant

Be Informed: Out-of-Date Approaches for Shrinking Nodules

There is a lot of out-of-date information regarding thyroid nodules. Your physician may be using outdated protocols, and even authoritative websites or books may provide obsolete information. To treat thyroid nodules, many physicians still use thyroid hormone (levothyroxine) in slightly higher than normal amounts to keep the TSH low and "suppress" the nodules. *This approach is more than twenty years out of date.* This practice was originally intended to discriminate between benign nodules that were expected to shrink with treatment and potentially malignant nodules that would continue to grow with treatment. Unfortunately, a large number of studies over the years have clearly shown that benign nodules will spontaneously shrink or grow regardless of whether thyroid hormone is given. For this reason, the treatment plan should be based on the results of the biopsy, not on a plan of thyroid hormone suppression therapy. If your doctor gives you thyroid hormone to shrink your nodule, it's time to find a new physician.

and stems from these epithelial cells, it's referred to as an adeno-carcinoma. This often applies to thyroid cancer, although the term doesn't describe what kind of thyroid cancer you have. The types of thyroid cancer include papillary thyroid cancer, follicular cancer, Hurthle cell cancer, anaplastic thyroid cancer, or medullary thyroid cancer (see Chapter 6 for specific information on each type of thyroid cancer). Very rarely, the malignant tumor is not a thyroid tumor, but one that has spread from another organ, such as the lung, breast, or kidney.

If the nodule is more than 1.0 cm (0.4 in.) in diameter, the surgeon should perform a total thyroidectomy. If the nodule is smaller, then the surgeon should remove half of the thyroid gland, pending the results of the final pathology. If the cancer is found to be anything larger or more extensive than a spot of papillary cancer (called a single focus) that is 1.0 cm (0.4 in.) or less or if it is any other type of thyroid cancer, then the surgeon should remove the rest of the gland during a second surgery.

Indeterminate or Suspicious Thyroid Nodules

With some nodules, the cytologist cannot find enough proof to suggest a thyroid cancer, nor do these nodule have the characteristics to prove they are benign, either. At least one-fifth of nodules classified as suspicious are proven to be thyroid cancer when a pathologist evaluates the thyroid gland after it is surgically removed.

When a nodule is defined as suspicious or indeterminate, there is no known test, short of surgery, that will determine completely whether it is cancer. For this reason, the most appropriate approach to a nodule with this classification is to have a surgeon remove the half of the gland containing the nodule, *not* just the nodule. If the surgeon finds definitive evidence of cancer during the surgery, then it's appropriate to remove the entire thyroid gland at once. If the pathologist finds that the indeterminate nodule is actually a thyroid cancer after surgery (when he or she reviews the slides later on), then a second surgery is needed to remove the rest of the thyroid gland.

If the surgery reveals that the nodule is benign, then there is no need for further thyroid surgery. You may, however, need to take

Be Informed: Beware Thyroid "Nodulectomy"

When it comes to evaluating thyroid nodules, any doctor who suggests surgical removal of the thyroid nodule without removing the complete half of the gland with the nodule is not competent to handle your thyroid nodule. This approach is considered substandard surgical care for several reasons. If the nodule is thyroid cancer, all further care requires that the entire thyroid gland must be surgically removed before any additional treatment can be given. In addition, many thyroid cancers are multifocal, meaning that many individual tumors are present at different places in the thyroid gland. This is not visible to the naked eye of the surgeon, so the entire lobe needs to be assessed for additional tumors. And finally, if a thyroid-ectomy is needed, the nodulectomy will make complications of thyroid surgery more likely because scarring from the original surgery can obscure key landmarks inside the neck that help the surgeon to avoid complications.

levothyroxine to compensate for the missing half of the thyroid gland, as one lobe may not be enough to make the right amount of thyroid hormone.

Follicular Neoplasia: Maybe Cancer, Maybe Not

Some thyroid nodules that are classified as indeterminate or suspicious fall into a category called follicular neoplasia. These nodules could be either benign follicular adenomas or follicular thyroid cancers. The only way to distinguish the benign adenoma from the cancer is by having the half of the thyroid gland containing the nodule surgically removed and carefully analyzed by a pathologist. For this reason, it's usually a good practice to request a second opinion from an outside expert thyroid pathologist, particularly when a benign follicular adenoma is diagnosed.

Who Should Be Screened for Thyroid Nodules?

In the 1940s and 1950s, many conditions were treated with external beam radiation therapy (EBRT) in the belief that it was therapeutic. We now know these therapies were potentially harmful. For example, some physicians believed that Sudden Infant Death Syndrome could be treated by x-ray therapy of the middle of the chest or that bad acne lesions or recurrent tonsil infections would be helped by EBRT. In other cases, there were clearly therapeutic uses similar to today's use of EBRT for Hodgkin's disease and other childhood cancers. But all of these treatments resulted in radiation exposures to the thyroid gland.

We now know that this practice predisposed exposed children to the development of thyroid cancer as adults. The risk for development of thyroid cancer seems to be greater the younger the child was when treated, with the greatest risk to those who were treated under five years of age. Those who were treated as older children are also at risk, although this diminishes considerably when the person was exposed when they were older than eighteen. This risk is not evident with the lower exposures associated with diagnostic x-ray tests, such as chest x-rays, simple CAT scans, dental films, or x-rays for broken bones.

Aside from EBRT, nuclear fallout usually contains radioactive iodine isotopes that carry radiation directly to the thyroid gland if they enter the body. Recent reports from the National Cancer Institute in the United States suggest that thousands of people have been placed at risk for developing thyroid cancer from their exposure to radioactive fallout from above-ground atomic testing in the 1950s and 1960s. This has been particularly noted in people exposed to fallout in the Marshall Islands during testing in 1954. This association of nuclear fallout with thyroid cancer was first recognized in the survivors of the atomic bombs dropped on Hiroshima and Nagasaki during World War II. Peacetime exposures have usually been seen during accidents at nuclear power plants. The most dramatic example was the explosion of the Chernobyl reactor in Belarus in 1986. A precipitous rise in thyroid cancer among children exposed to radioactive fallout (some while in their mother's womb) removed any doubt concerning this risk. Even more notable was the absence of thyroid cancer in nearby Polish children who had been given potassium iodide pills to prevent them from absorbing the radioactive iodine fallout in an otherwise similar exposure.

Were You Exposed to Radiation?

Knowing whether you were exposed to radiation as a child is the first concern. Clearly, you won't know about exposure as an infant unless you ask your parents or have access to all your medical records. Although inappropriate uses of EBRT should have ended by the 1960s, several people were given such treatment as recently as 1978. There are maps documenting the estimated sites and dates of radioactive fallout exposure in the United States during the 1950s, although other factors are involved. For example, the only significant exposures in many regions are thought to have occurred in people drinking milk from their own dairy cows who ate contaminated grass. Milk from local dairies in the same region, however, was not likely to be contaminated because the extra time it took for this milk to be collected, processed, packaged, and sold resulted in the loss of most of the short-lived radioactive iodine isotopes.

It is interesting to note that exposure to radioactive iodine, given as a diagnostic dose to perform a thyroid scan or given as a larger dose to treat Graves' disease or ATN, does *not* put you at risk for the development of thyroid cancer. It's been observed (and theorized) that the radiation dose to the thyroid from a radioactive iodine scan is too low to cause this risk; conversely, in the case of radioactive iodine treatment doses, they are too high to cause the risk because they are high enough to kill thyroid cancer cells outright. Both perceived and actual risks from radioactive iodine are often very different (see Chapter 9).

If you find that your thyroid gland was exposed to radiation at any time, particularly when you were a child, it's crucial to perform a thyroid self-examination on a regular basis. If your thyroid gland is difficult to feel, request a baseline thyroid ultrasound examination. The ultrasound frequently finds tiny nodules that are too small to be of significance; however, any nodule exceeding 1.0 cm (0.4 in.) in diameter discovered by any technique should trigger the investigation process discussed earlier. In the event that the nodule is suspicious—it keeps growing in spite of benign or indeterminate biopsy results—you should seek out a surgeon to remove the half of the thyroid with the nodule so it can be analyzed more thoroughly. If you have multiple nodules, this may even be a good opportunity to remove the entire thyroid gland.

Some physicians advise people with a history of radiation exposure to take thyroid hormone medication in high enough amounts to suppress TSH levels. This does not reduce the risk of thyroid cancer, although it does seem to reduce the number of nodules that develop. Using thyroid hormone medication may provide some advantage in reducing the number of times that nodules need to be assessed, but it is not clear whether it's useful for everyone in this situation. Certainly, it should be considered as a treatment if benign nodules are found.

6

Thyroid Cancer

A Beginner's Guide

THYROID CANCER STILL remains a rare cancer, accounting for about 2 percent of cancers in people of all ages and 4 percent of cancers in children. Nevertheless, thyroid cancer is now ranked as the fastest-rising cancer in men and women, topping the rate of increase in lung and breast cancers. Women outnumber men in developing thyroid cancer by three to one; women account for 75 percent of new cases of thyroid cancer; and 58 percent of deaths from thyroid cancer occur in women. In 2004 an estimated 5,900 men developed thyroid cancer, compared to 17,700 women; in the same year, around 620 deaths from thyroid cancer occurred in men and 850 deaths occurred in women. This statistical imbalance may have something to do with the fact that while thyroid cancers are seen much more frequently in women, they seem to be more lethal in men. It is currently not known why these gender differences exist.

What Causes Thyroid Cancer?

In most cases of thyroid cancer, there is no known cause. As discussed in Chapter 5, people most at risk for thyroid cancer are those who were exposed to radiation or radioactive iodine from nuclear fallout. When the healthy thyroid gland is exposed to radioactive iodine, the cells of the thyroid gland can develop breaks in their chromosomes, which can cause cancer. Several studies have confirmed high rates of thyroid cancer in certain areas or populations. One study, published in 1997 by the National Cancer Institute, looked at health risks of radioactive fallout released at the Nevada Test Site from 1951 through 1958. The study concluded that people living in the midwestern regions of North America were more at risk for thyroid cancer, particularly if they were children during the testing. Reports of high rates of thyroid cancer are also coming in from Hanford, Washington, where residents were exposed to fallout from the Hanford nuclear facility, which produced plutonium for nuclear weapons from 1944 through 1957. In the Marshall Islands in the South Pacific, as a result of atomic bomb testing at Bikini Atoll in 1954, thyroid cancer occurs 100 times more frequently than in the unexposed population.

The nuclear accident at the Chernobyl atomic power station on April 26, 1986, exposed millions of people with healthy thyroid glands to excessive levels of radioactive iodine. People living within a 30-kilometer radius of the accident inhaled the radioactive iodine, while people living outside the 30-kilometer radius ingested the radioactive iodine. For reasons not quite understood, potassium iodide tablets (thyroid blocking agents) weren't distributed to the public by the appropriate government agencies except in Poland. In Belarus, Russia, and the Ukraine, there currently appears to be a 100-fold increase in the incidence of thyroid cancer in children and an increase of thyroid cancer in adults. For example, one study out of the Ukraine found that between 1981 and 1985, the number of new cases of thyroid cancer in children aged zero to fourteen totaled 25. But between 1986 and 1994, the number of new cases of thyroid cancer in this age group totaled 210, with peak periods in 1992 and 1993.

In other cases, radiation to the head and neck area from external beam radiation therapy, or high-dose x-rays, during childhood or adolescence can cause thyroid cancer to develop later in life, as discussed in Chapter 5.

Inherited Thyroid Cancer

There is one type of thyroid cancer in which a genetic mutation, called an autosomal dominant genetic disorder, is passed from either parent to his or her child. In these instances, there is a 50 percent chance that a parent will pass on the mutation to his or her child. If a person has even one gene with the genetic mutation for this type of cancer, called familial medullary thyroid cancer (FMTC), the chance that he or she will develop it is almost 100 percent. Individuals who come from a family with this genetic disorder (who are called *kindreds*) have extremely high odds of carrying the gene. FMTC is discussed in more detail later in this chapter.

Some forms of medullary thyroid cancer are spontaneous, rather than inherited. Genetic screening can be used to determine whether you have the mutation for FMTC. A prophylactic thyroidectomy should be performed as soon as the mutation is discovered since there is no good treatment for medullary thyroid cancer, unlike the more common forms of thyroid cancer, regardless of how young the child is. Age two is the recommended age if the gene is discovered earlier than three.

Some unusual families seem to have more cases of papillary cancers than chance would account for. The genetic basis of these cases has not yet been discovered.

Signs of Thyroid Cancer

Thyroid cancer is typically discovered during the evaluation of a thyroid nodule. It is also sometimes found after a tumor is discovered elsewhere in the body, such as in the lungs or in a bone, with the biopsy of this tumor eventually pointing out the thyroid as the source of the cancer. It's important to recognize the signs of thyroid cancer, particularly if your thyroid has been exposed to radiation. Often the signs are not that obvious, but they can include:

- A hard and painless lump anywhere on your neck; this is the most common first sign of thyroid cancer
- A thyroid nodule that continues to enlarge
- Difficulty swallowing food or liquids
- A change in your voice or hoarseness (this may indicate that the cancer is spreading beyond the thyroid gland)

- Pain in your neck tissues, jawbone, or, less commonly, ear
- Sleep apnea, a sleep disorder characterized by interrupted breathing, that has come on suddenly; this is very rare, but there have been cases in which thyroid cancer patients have been falsely diagnosed with sleep apnea when, in fact, a growing thyroid tumor was present that caused difficulty breathing

Pete's Story: Son of an FMTC Kindred

For as long as I can remember, cancer has been a part of our family. I never knew what kind of cancer killed my grandfather, my three uncles, my one aunt, my four cousins, and my dad. My grandfather married three times and had three different families, so I have many, many cousins. I got a call from one of my cousins (who I have never met) about two years ago. She told me that she was "managing a family problem with a genetic cancer." She had been diagnosed with thyroid cancer but told that there was no good treatment for it. She was told that she had a genetic mutation that caused the cancer and that she needed to tell her family members about it so they could have surgery. She suspected that this gene was passed down the line from our common grandfather (her mother's father). There have been about forty-eight people in our family that have had their thyroids removed. The three families my grandfather created have eleven children who are his direct offspring; most of them have three or more children. My grandfather was also one of thirteen children, and there are still great-aunts and -uncles who are contacting their children and grandchildren after they tested positive. I had my thyroid surgery recently; when they removed it, it had already started to grow cancer, which was confined to the thyroid. One of my children also tested positive and will soon have her thyroid removed. Our family owes a great debt to my cousin, and this cancer has helped our family unite. My cousin also organized a large family reunion so we could all meet and compare notes, but she died shortly after.

Types of Thyroid Cancer

This section discusses the types of thyroid cancer. Treatment is discussed in a separate section.

Papillary Thyroid Cancer

Papillary tumors account for roughly 80 percent of all thyroid cancers, and it is usually treatable. The frightening aspect of papillary thyroid cancer is that it tends to spread, usually to the lymph nodes in the neck. This creates a higher recurrence rate but not usually a higher mortality rate. The ten-year survival rate remains at 80 to 90 percent, meaning that ten years after this diagnosis, 80 to 90 percent of people diagnosed with papillary thyroid cancer are still alive.

Most people with papillary cancer will not experience a metastasis, or spread of the cancer, beyond the neck. But sometimes there can be what's called a distant metastasis to the lungs or bones. Papillary cancer tends to strike most often in people ages thirty through fifty, and it develops in women three times more frequently than men. As is the case with most cancer, the smaller the tumor, the better the news. Thyroid cancers that are less than 0.5 in. are considered to be the most treatable. Most thyroid cancers caused by radiation exposure are papillary cancers.

Tall Cell Papillary Cancer

Once you get papillary cancer cells under a microscope, things get a little more complicated because there are variations of papillary cancers. There are subtypes of thyroid cancer tumors and there are some cell variants that can make the normally slow-growing papillary a little more aggressive. The tall cell variant of papillary thyroid cancer spreads more rapidly and has a greater chance of losing the ability to suck up iodine. Because it spreads faster, recurrence is more likely, requiring more vigilant follow-up than the usual papillary cancer. More assertive surgery and follow-up care is also required, considering the risk of metastasis.

Follicular Thyroid Cancer

Roughly 10 percent of all thyroid cancers are purely follicular. This type of thyroid cancer does not commonly occur as a direct result of radiation exposure. Follicular cancer tends to strike most in people aged forty to sixty and, again, it occurs three times more often in women than men. Age is the most important factor in deciding how treatable a case of follicular thyroid cancer will be. Follicular thyroid cancer tends to be less aggressive in people under forty years than in people over forty; this is because it responds better to radioactive iodine therapy in younger people. Follicular thyroid cancer also tends to invade the veins and arteries of the thyroid gland, as well as distant organs, such as the lungs, bones, brain, liver, bladder, and skin. Only about 15 percent of follicular cancers spread to the lymph nodes—a very different picture than papillary cancers. As dismal as it sounds, the overall cure rate for purely follicular thyroid cancer is almost 95 percent in people under forty. After that, the cure rate depends greatly on the staging, discussed later in this chapter.

Hurthle Cell Cancer: A Close Relative

Hurthle cell thyroid cancer, or oncocytic thyroid cancer, is a type of follicular thyroid cancer. This is an unusual type of tumor that's less common than follicular cancer, making up only 4 percent of all thyroid cancers. Most people who develop Hurthle cell thyroid cancer are in their midfifties and older—about ten years older than those with the follicular type. Hurthle cell cancer doesn't tend to spread to the lymph nodes, but it can sprout again in the same place or spread to the lungs or bones. It may take years for Hurthle cell cancers to grow and do much damage. The cure rate relates, as with follicular cancers, to the staging.

Uncommon Types of Thyroid Cancer

There are some less common types of thyroid cancer that I will discuss only briefly here.

Medullary Thyroid Cancer

Medullary thyroid cancer (MTC), which accounts for fewer than one out of ten cases of thyroid cancer found in the United States each year, can be spontaneous or inherited (FMTC, discussed earlier in this chapter). Medullary thyroid cancer involves the parafollicular cell (C cell), which does not make thyroid hormone or take up iodine. Therefore, radioactive iodine cannot be used as a treatment for this aggressive type of cancer. Surgery is the main treatment for this cancer, although experimental trials may be used when the cancer is advanced.

The best way to treat MTC is through prevention. If you are diagnosed with MTC, you should have the genetic test to see if you have the inherited form; if so, your children, siblings, and other family members should be tested too. If they have the mutation, then they have a virtually 100 percent chance of developing this cancer at some point; a prophylactic thyrodectomy can prevent this cancer from developing or from spreading if caught early.

Unresponsive Aggressive Thyroid Cancer Tumors

Anaplastic thyroid cancer is a wildly undifferentiated cancer that accounts for only about three hundred cases of thyroid cancer per year in the United States. Papillary or follicular thyroid cancers may become anaplastic—a very aggressive, untreatable form of thyroid cancer—if they are not treated. There are also cases where papillary or follicular thyroid cancers are unresponsive to treatment and can become aggressive tumors.

Staging and Spreading

While people can be diagnosed with the same kind of thyroid cancer, their treatments will depend on the stage, or phase, of the cancer. Staging systems are not useful in predicting the outcomes of individual cases of thyroid cancer; they're mainly used as a way to predict general trends in thyroid cancer in large groups of patients. Most thyroid cancers have four stage classifications that basically answer the question, "Where has it spread?"

Papillary Stages

For papillary cancer, Stage I means that the cancer is confined to the thyroid gland in either one lobe or both lobes. Stage II in people under forty-five years means the cancer has spread beyond the thyroid; in people over forty-five, it means that the cancer may still be confined to the thyroid, but is larger than 0.5 in. Stage III means the cancer has spread beyond the thyroid to surrounding lymph nodes but has not gone beyond the neck. If you're younger than forty-five, you won't get to Stage III. Stage IV is also only seen in people over forty-five years and means the cancer has spread to distant organs, such as the lungs or the bones.

Follicular Stages

For follicular thyroid cancer, Stage I means the cancer is confined to the thyroid, in either one lobe or both. Stage II in people under forty-five means the cancer has spread beyond the thyroid gland; in people over forty-five it means a larger tumor, about 0.5 in., confined to the thyroid. Stage III is seen only in people over forty-five and means the cancer has spread outside the thyroid, possibly to the lymph nodes, but not beyond the neck. Stage IV, also seen only in people over forty-five, means the cancer has spread to distant organs, such as the lungs or bones.

Differentiated Versus Undifferentiated

No matter how old you are, what size the tumor is, or how far it has spread, the defining and most critical feature of thyroid cancer is whether it is differentiated or undifferentiated. Differentiated cancer cells are cells that retain the *functional* features of normal thyroid cells. These features include having functional thyroid-stimulating hormone receptors, so that TSH stimulates these cells to grow and lack of TSH causes them to "sleep"; responding to TSH, in that they have the ability to "suck up" iodine and to produce thyroglobulin (Tg); and a generally slow rate of growth (in comparison to many other types of cancers). Thyroid cancer cells that are well or moderately differentiated tend to respond well to treatment with surgery and radioactive iodine.

Cancer cells that are either poorly differentiated or undifferentiated do not have the functional features of a normal thyroid cell. This means that you cannot use radioactive iodine scans to find them or treat them. When these cancer cells spread beyond the neck to other parts of the body, they become difficult or impossible to treat. New treatments are needed for these poorly differentiated thyroid cancers.

Treating Common Types of Thyroid Cancer

For the majority of papillary and follicular thyroid cancers and their variants, treatment always involves surgery, but there are different kinds of surgeries. A partial thyroidectomy removes some or most of the thyroid gland. When only one lobe, or one half, of the thyroid gland is removed, it is called a lobectomy. A partial thyroidectomy is not synonymous with a lobectomy, since a partial thyroidectomy can mean anything from a tiny bit of a thyroid gland removed to 90 percent of the thyroid gland being removed. A total thyroidectomy excises the entire thyroid gland. A neck dissection removes lymph nodes in the neck that may contain cancer. Beyond surgery, there are options for further treatment.

- **Radioactive iodine (RAI) therapy.** The effectiveness of this treatment depends on the stage of your cancer and on whether you have a more aggressive form of cancer, such as follicular or tall cell papillary. RAI therapy involves taking a capsule or liquid form of RAI. Because the thyroid absorbs iodine, any differentiated thyroid cancer cells, such as papillary and follicular, should absorb the radioactive iodine, which will kill them. RAI is discussed more in Chapter 9.
- **External beam radiation therapy.** Generally reserved for a more advanced stage or for aggressive types of thyroid cancer that do not take up radioactive iodine, this treatment involves using high-dose x-rays or other similar high-energy rays to kill cancer cells. This is an option that probably won't be presented unless your thyroid cancer progresses in spite of surgery and RAI.
- **Hormone therapy.** When your thyroid gland is removed, you will be hypothyroid (see Chapter 2). You will therefore need to be on thyroid hormone to function at all, and you will also need to be on a TSH suppression dosage (see Chapter 10 on thyroid hormone).
- **Beta-blockers.** If you have symptoms of thyrotoxicosis from TSH-suppressive dosages of thyroid hormone, you may need to be put on a beta-blocker (see Chapter 3).

Typical Treatment Plans

Papillary thyroid cancers that are 1 cm or less in size (less than 0.4 in.), exist as a single tumor within the thyroid gland, and show no evidence of any spread to the neck or elsewhere, can be treated with surgery alone (usually removal of the half of the thyroid where the tumor was—a lobectomy). These small papillary cancers do not require radioactive iodine scans or treatments. Many physicians will have you take thyroid hormone to keep your TSH level slightly less than normal, although you may not be told to take any thyroid hormone at all.

All other papillary cancers and all follicular thyroid cancers of any size require a total (or near total) removal of the thyroid gland and removal of any lymph nodes in the neck that are likely to contain a tumor. (See the section on thyroidectomy later in this chapter.) This is followed by radioactive iodine therapy (see Chapter 9), with routine RAI scans and blood tests to measure thyroglobulin (Tg). You will also need to follow a low-iodine diet for both RAI therapy or scans (see Chapter 11 for more information on diet and dietary iodine).

What You Should Know About Thyroidectomy

When you have your thyroid removed, as long as the piece of thyroid gland that's been left behind is minimal (less than 2 g by weight), it is considered a total or near-total thyroidectomy. There's no reason for a surgeon to purposely remove only part of a thyroid lobe or to remove the cancerous nodule by itself unless the tumor is invading the neck so aggressively that he or she cannot do more surgery safely.

Total thyroidectomy versus partial thyroidectomy is an extremely controversial issue right now with thyroid surgeons and endocrinologists. Partial thyroidectomy is generally not recommended and is only acceptable if you have a single papillary cancer nodule of less than 1 cm with no evidence of spread to any other area. This is because such small papillary cancers will rarely cause further problems after such surgery. Otherwise, the only appropriate choice should be between a total thyroidectomy and a near-total thyroidectomy. This is because most cancers have a reasonably high chance of having spread to the opposite side of the thyroid gland or beyond the thyroid gland into the neck or more distant sites.

Very experienced thyroid surgeons who perform many thyroid surgeries each year (more than twenty-five) feel capable of doing total thyroidectomies. Surgeons with fewer cases or less experience often want to leave small pieces of the thyroid gland behind (usually near the vocal cord nerves or parathyroid glands), a near-total thyroidectomy.

Risks of Surgery: Why the Surgeon Needs to Be Experienced

In total thyroidectomy surgery with a very experienced thyroid surgeon, there's roughly a 2 percent chance of permanent damage to the nerves of the voice box or to the parathyroid glands. However, considering that only 2 percent of the population gets thyroid cancer, 2 percent is not such a low percentage to thyroid cancer patients.

Be Informed: Which Type of Thyroidectomy?

Sometimes people with biopsy-proven thyroid cancer are recommended for a partial thyroidectomy. This is not recommended and is a sign that the surgeon may not be that experienced with thyroid removal. The majority of thyroid cancer patients will have a total thyroidectomy and modified neck dissection, which involves removing all the thyroid gland and any nearby lymph nodes that are cancerous.

Partial thyroidectomy is reserved for people with small papillary cancers (under 1 cm in diameter) and can involve a few types of procedures. One procedure, a lobectomy, involves removing one lobe. Another procedure, called a lobectomy and isthmusectomy, involves removing one lobe and the isthmus, which is the bridge of tissue linking the lobes of the thyroid gland together (like the horizontal line in an H). A near-total thyroidectomy or subtotal thyroidectomy removes the tumor from the cancerous side of the gland, as well as the isthmus and most of the other lobe.

Many thyroid cancer experts support that a total thyroidectomy should be performed for most cancers because it is necessary for proper treatment and accurate long-term follow-up.

When you're considering your treatment plan, you'll have to weigh that 2 percent risk against the fact that thyroid cancer patients whose papillary tumors are greater than 1 cm and who have a total thyroid-ectomy followed by radioactive iodine therapy and thyroid suppression have a significantly lower recurrence rate of their cancers. In addition, the less normal thyroid tissue left in your body, the greater the benefit of radioactive iodine therapy after surgery. RAI therapy is an important way to eradicate the thyroid cells that are frequently left behind after surgery, which are all potentially cancerous tissue. But if there's half a thyroid gland still left inside you, the radioactive iodine will probably wind up in the intact lobe, causing thyroiditis, which happens about 60 percent of the time. The bottom line is that the more thyroid tissue there is left inside you, the less effective the treatment and follow-up to the cancer may be. Despite potential problems, it may be worth having a total thyroidectomy to absolutely minimize your risk of recurrence and optimize your care.

Repeat thyroid surgery also may involve working through previous scar tissue, which can take longer and may involve more complications. Having another surgery performed in the same site as a previous thyroid surgery makes having problems with damaged parathyroid glands and paralyzed vocal cords far more likely. Thus, you'd never want a surgeon to remove part of a thyroid lobe, putting you at risk for another surgery on that same side. If the risks of complications are 2 percent for experienced thyroid surgeons, these risks are greater for less experienced surgeons.

Vocal Cord Nerve Damage

The vocal cord nerves on both sides pass near (or into) the thyroid gland. If one nerve is damaged during surgery, then the vocal cord it connects to becomes paralyzed, causing a hoarse or weak voice. Sometimes the tumor itself causes this problem by eating its way into these nerves. If both nerves become damaged, then you may need to have a hole made in the windpipe (a tracheostomy) to permit you to breathe.

The most experienced surgeons are least likely to damage the vocal cords; however, this is a known risk of this surgery and should be carefully explained to you before you consent to the surgery. It's good practice to ask the surgeon about the frequency with which these problems have occurred in his or her other patients and about his or her own experience and training in this surgery.

Numbness and Nerve Damage

Thyroid surgery frequently involves cutting nerve endings in the neck area, which can leave parts of your neck and shoulder area numb. Some thyroid cancer survivors have even had numbness around ear lobes or the tongue. It can take years for these nerve endings to grow back. Each person will have different types of numbness that can often be helped through massage or acupuncture (see Chapter 12). Sometimes you can still feel itches on the numb regions but lack the ability to scratch them. This can be maddening but may be controlled through creams recommended by a dermatologist.

Hypothyroidism

After surgery, you will be permanently hypothyroid unless you take thyroid hormone. This is considered not as a risk but rather as an outcome of the surgery. See Chapter 2 for more information on the symptoms of hypothyroidism and Chapter 10 for more on thyroid hormone.

Hypoparathyroidism

The most common risk of thyroid surgery is damage to the parathyroid glands. These four tiny glands are found near the thyroid gland and can be damaged or mistaken by the surgeon for lymph nodes. They make parathyroid hormone (PTH), which controls the calcium level in your body, telling the kidney to keep calcium from going out in the urine and enhancing the activation of vitamin D to absorb more calcium from the intestines. If all four parathyroid glands are damaged, the resulting loss of PTH, called hypoparathyroidism, causes the kidneys to lose calcium in the urine and decreases their ability to absorb more calcium. The result is that calcium levels plummet. This causes numbness or tingling sensations around the lips, numbness or tingling of the hands or feet, muscle cramps, twitching, and sometimes seizures. If the parathyroid glands are merely bruised from the surgery, the resulting hypocalcemia (low calcium) will be temporary, lasting from days to weeks. If the parathyroid glands have been accidentally removed or their blood supply disrupted during the surgery, the loss of PTH can be permanent. Although severe PTH disturbances can be detected by obtaining a calcium level, an ionized calcium level is the most sensitive test for this.

Treatment of hypoparathyroidism entails taking high doses of activated forms of vitamin D, along with sufficient calcium pills to maintain the ionized calcium within the low end of the normal range. Vitamin D analogs (calcitriol, dihydrotachysterol, or vitamin D2) cause the intestines to absorb sufficient amounts of the calcium pills to offset the calcium losses through the kidney.

Follow-Up Scans and Tests

Thyroid cancer patients will need to go for regular follow-up scans involving radioactive iodine. Preparation for these scans includes being made hypothyroid or taking a drug called Thyrogen (see Chapter 9), as well as following the low-iodine diet prior to a radioactive iodine scan or treatment (see Chapter 11).

Thyroglobulin Testing

Thyroglobulin (Tg) is a protein that is made only by thyroid cells or thyroid cancer cells. No other part of the body can make this special protein. Usually, thyroid or thyroid cancer cells release this protein into the blood, making it possible to measure it in a blood sample. Since there is no other source of thyroglobulin, once the thyroid gland has been completely removed by surgery and its remnants destroyed by radioactive iodine, there should be no measurable thyroglobulin left in the blood. Thus, the presence of measurable thyroglobulin indicates the presence of thyroid cancer. (Note that it's important not to confuse the thyroglobulin level with the thyroglobulin antibody level or a thyroxine-binding globulin level, both of which are unrelated and often confused by patients *and* doctors for the thyroglobulin level.)

You should have a blood test for thyroglobulin at least every six months. This will only be an accurate indicator of a thyroid cancer recurrence if you've had a total thyroidectomy followed by radioactive iodine therapy. The thyroglobulin test (Tg test) is more accurate when your TSH level is not suppressed; the usual method is to perform Tg tests while you are hypothyroid or taking Thyrogen (see Chapter 9), when appropriate. Some physicians believe that selected patients with low risks of thyroid cancer recurrence may be evaluated with Thyrogen-stimulated Tg testing only after their scans are clean and they're having regular Tg tests with results that are so low as to be undetectable.

It's important to account for cancers that may have lost the ability to make thyroglobulin or take up radioactive iodine. This can be assessed with additional imaging tests (such as MRI scans or CT scans without contrast dye), as well as MIBI scans, PET scans, or nuclear scans using radioactive thallium.

Around one-quarter or more of thyroid cancer patients, particularly women, have immune systems that produce antibodies against their own thyroglobulin. The reasons for this are not clearly understood and they do not directly influence your health; however, this can make thyroglobulin testing difficult or even impossible. This is because these antibodies interfere with the blood test for thyroglobulin performed in the laboratory and prevent the thyroglobulin level in your blood from being accurately measured. Thus, it is standard practice to measure both the thyroglobulin level and the thyroglobulin antibody level each time a thyroglobulin assessment is made. If the thyroglobulin antibody level is undetectable, then the measured thyroglobulin level may be considered reliable. If thyroglobulin antibody level is above the normal values for the laboratory, then you cannot rely upon the thyroglobulin level to confirm that you are free from persistent thyroid cancer.

Thyroid Hormone Suppression Therapy

If you've had papillary or follicular thyroid cancer, you'll be placed on a suppression dosage of thyroid hormone. Any microscopic bit of thyroid cancer in your body may be stimulated by thyroid-stimulating hormone. The trick is to find a high enough dosage to suppress your TSH levels; this means that blood tests will show that you have higher free T4 readings than hypothyroid patients who are merely taking thyroid hormone to keep themselves in the normal range. TSH suppression can be accomplished without causing you to become thyro-toxic (see Chapter 3). Thyroid hormone is discussed in more detail in Chapter 10.

Treating Recurrence

Recurrence of papillary or follicular thyroid cancer often means another round of RAI scans and treatments, perhaps further surgery, and possibly even external beam radiation therapy. If there's a distant spread of papillary or follicular cancer to other organs, you may be offered something known as dosimetry, a procedure in which the highest possible dose of RAI is calculated according to a meticulous course of measurements and calculations using a tracer dose of radio-active iodine in you.

7

Complications, Other Conditions, and Comorbidities

When Other Stuff Happens, Too

COMPLICATIONS OF THYROID disease may arise as a direct result of either autoimmune thyroid disease, as is the case with Graves'-related eye problems, or heart problems. Other natural conditions, such as normal stress, aging, and menopause, may mask or complicate thyroid disease. There are also comorbidities, or coexisting diseases. Pre-existing cardiovascular disease, depression, and sleep disorders may worsen or aggravate your thyroid problem, or mask symptoms of thyroid problems. (Obesity is another comorbidity that is discussed in Chapter 11.) There is also what I call the autoimmune collection package, in which several autoimmune diseases may strike at once, creating chaos. This chapter helps to untangle the other things going on in your body and life that may affect thyroid disease or become a barrier to diagnosing it.

Thyroid Eye Disease

A frustrating complication associated with autoimmune thyroid disorders is thyroid eye disease (TED). Thyroid eye disease tends to strike people with Graves'-related hyperthyroidism (see Chapter 3) and sometimes even those suffering from Hashimoto's disease (see Chapter 2). In clinical circles, TED is known by several different names: Graves' ophthalmopathy (GO), thyroid-associated ophthalmopathy, and, infrequently, dysthyroid orbitopathy. (The prefix *ophthalmo-* means "eyes," while *-pathy* means "disease.") This disease is characterized by bulging, watery eyes, a condition known as exophthalmos.

A common symptom of excessive thyroid hormone is lid retraction. Here, your upper eyelids can retract slightly and expose more of the whites of your eyes. The lid retraction creates a rather dramatic staring look. This specific symptom is related to the excessive activation of the adrenaline system from thyrotoxicosis and can be seen in nonautoimmune thyrotoxicosis. It will improve with beta-blockers. It's different from the actual bulging of the eyes, called proptosis, which only occurs in autoimmune thyroid disease. The lid retraction will usually improve when the hyperthyroidism is treated. This is not always the case with proptosis, as many people also have bulging of their eyeballs from underlying TED, which seems to persist long after the hyperthyroidism ends.

When TED is associated with the hyperthyroidism of Graves' disease, the eye problems can be far more severe. At least 50 percent of all Graves' disease patients suffer from obvious TED. At one time, only those with noticeable changes to the eyes were considered to have TED, but more sophisticated methods of diagnosis reveal that eye changes are present in almost all Graves' disease patients, even though symptoms may not be noticeable.

It is believed that the autoimmune antibodies that develop in Graves' disease cause TED. For some reason, the same proteins in your thyroid cells and your eye muscle cells react to the antithyroid antibodies that occur with Graves' disease. Treatment of the thyroid does not usually help the eyes, which continues to frustrate TED sufferers.

Smoking and Thyroid Eye Disease

Smokers are far more likely to suffer from severe TED than nonsmokers, although stress seems to aggravate the condition, too. As for smoking, the link between smoking and thyroid eye disease is so strong that thyroid specialists believe smokers with Graves' disease can probably count on developing TED. The following facts are known about smoking and Graves' disease:

- Smoking worsens the course of Graves' disease and its severity.
- Smoking increases the likelihood that a person with Graves' disease will have significant TED.
- People with such severe TED that they need steroid treatments or radiation treatment to their eyes will not respond as well to these treatments if they smoke.
- Ex-smokers do not have such risk for the development and worsening of their Graves' disease, suggesting a value to stopping any smoking as soon as possible.

The Symptoms of Thyroid Eye Disease

The most common eye changes caused by TED are bulging and double vision. These symptoms are caused by inflammation of the eye tissues:

Randy's Story: Smoking and Thyroid Eye Disease

Several months before my Graves' disease was diagnosed, I started having trouble with my eyes. They felt irritated and gritty. When I couldn't close them all the way, I saw an eye doctor. He was the one who sent me to my thyroid doctor, telling me that thyroid eye disease is not as common in men. So now I had this "woman's disease"—that made me feel worse. My eyes were bulging so badly, I needed to wear sunglasses most of the time to hide them; people were beginning to stare at me. My thyroid doctor diagnosed me with Graves' disease. He asked me if I was a smoker. When I said I was, he told me that all the Graves' patients who smoke get the eye problems like me and that if I quit, the eye problems might get better. I had to go into a nicotine withdrawal program and on antithyroid drugs at the same time.

the eyes become painful, red, and watery with a gritty feeling. Sensitivity to light, wind, or sun is also common. The grittiness and light sensitivity worsen with lid retraction, as the eyes are less protected by the eyelids from dust, wind, and infection.

Other symptoms include discomfort when looking up or to the side. And while some Graves' disease patients suffer from excessive watering of the eyes, many also suffer from excessive dryness. In rare and extreme cases, vision deteriorates as a result of too much pressure being placed on the optic nerve from the protruding eyeball.

The covering of the eye also becomes inflamed and swollen. The eyelids and the tissues around the eyes are swollen with fluid, and the eyeballs tend to bulge out of their sockets. Because of eye muscle damage or thickening, the eyes cannot move normally, resulting in blurred or double vision.

Interestingly, some people notice that TED symptoms worsen when their thyroid hormone levels are lower than normal. Because hypothyroidism causes bloating and fluid retention, this can exacerbate inflammation of the eyes, triggering TED symptoms such as dryness and grittiness. Many thyroid patients have ongoing disputes with their physicians over whether their TED flare-up is related to their thyroid condition. It may be. Since much is unknown about the relationship between TED and thyroid hormone levels, you do not have to accept your doctor's word.

During what's called the hot phase, or the initial active phase of TED, inflammation and swelling around and behind the eye are common. This phase lasts about six months, followed by the cold phase, in which the inflammation subsides and the visual changes are more noticeable.

In severe cases the swelling may be so bad that you will find it difficult to move your eye, and you may even develop ulcers on the cornea. This comes from constant exposure to the air because the eye is so swollen that the lids can't close to distribute the lubricating tears. In most cases both eyes are affected, but one may be worse than the other. You may also experience a phenomenon called lid lag, in which your upper lids are slow to move when you're looking down. Lid lag results from the effects of too much thyroid hormone and will go away if your thyroid hormone levels are lowered or you are treated with a beta-blocker medication.

Generally, the changes to the eyes reach a burnout period within a two-year time frame and then stop. Severe cases of TED can progress to blindness, even with proper intervention, but this is very rare. Sometimes the eyes get better by themselves, but often, after the burnout period, the eyes remain changed but do not get any worse. An ophthalmologist can measure the severity of the eye changes with an instrument called an exophthalmometer, which measures the degree to which the eyes protrude from the skull.

The Stages of Thyroid Eye Disease

In 80 percent of cases of Graves'-associated eye disease, symptoms of TED appear about a year or more before the symptoms of the Graves' disease itself. This, of course, can be very frustrating and may throw your doctor off the scent of thyroid disease altogether. When symptoms first appear, TED is said to be in its active, or initial, phase. This can last anywhere from eighteen to twenty-four months. During the active phase, you will experience the most dramatic eye changes, and it may not be necessary to treat the condition beyond symptom relief until the eyes reach their burnout phase. This means the eye problem will reach a "maximum change" point, after which they will probably remain changed but not worsen. On the other hand, a few people have a rapid worsening that requires steroid treatments or surgery or both.

Getting a Diagnosis

TED is frequently misdiagnosed as an allergy or pink eye (conjunctivitis). One easy way to confirm TED is to request that your thyroid be checked and also to request a thyroid-stimulating antibody test. Imaging tests such as computerized tomography (CT), ultrasound, or magnetic resonance imaging (MRI) may be used to view the orbit or eye tissues.

Treating Thyroid Eye Disease

You cannot treat TED if you don't know you have TED. In some cases, the eye symptoms may precede other signs of thyroid disease. In other cases, the eye symptoms may not appear until long after the thyroid disease is treated. So it is important to recognize that the symptoms of TED are related to thyroid disease in the first place before any effective treatments for TED can be planned. In cases where the eye symptoms appear before any signs of thyroid disease, a good doctor will try to discover reasons for the symptoms, and exclude other causes, such as tumors in the eye socket, which would be evaluated with an MRI or a CT scan. In some cases, when the hyperthyroidism is treated, the eyes tend to get better—even before burnout occurs. And TED in the absence of hyperthyroidism tends to be much easier to treat. If hyperthyroidism is treated with radioactive iodine, it may make TED worse.

Drug Treatments

The first step in treating TED is using artificial tears during the day and lubricating ointment at bedtime. If TED becomes worse, the next step is to prescribe prednisone, a steroid, which reduces swelling and inflammation causing the more severe TED symptoms. Steroids have numerous side effects, however, and you'll need to make an informed decision in balancing these side effects against the TED symptoms. The other problem with steroids is that once you go off of them, TED symptoms can resume and may even get worse.

Other Treatments

If you choose not to go on steroids, you can have radiation therapy, or you may be a candidate for a surgical procedure known as orbital decompression surgery. These treatments are very involved, beyond what can be covered here. Your doctor can help you determine if these options might be a good choice for you.

Depression or Anxiety: Could It Be My Thyroid?

If you look at the list of symptoms that comprise hypothyroidism (Chapter 2) and thyrotoxicosis (Chapter 3), many of them overlap and collide with symptoms of depression and anxiety. Both depression and anxiety can be a consequence of untreated hypothyroidism or thyrotoxicosis. The most common type of depression frequently associated with hypothyroidism is unipolar depression, which is characterized by one low or flat mood. This is distinct from bipolar depression, which is characterized by two moods, a higher mood and a lower mood, that typically cycle. A few symptoms of bipolar depression can sometimes be confused with thyrotoxicosis, but the exhaustion that accompanies thyrotoxicosis is not present in people with bipolar disorder.

Unipolar Depression and Hypothyroidism

Most cases of unipolar or major depression are caused by life circumstances and/or situations. For this reason, the term *situational depression* is used by mental health care experts to describe most cases of mild, moderate, or even severe unipolar depression. Examples of a life event include:

- Illness (including your thyroid disease)
- Loss of a loved one or a relationship
- Major life change
- Job loss or change
- Moving

Situational depression can also be triggered by the absence of change in your life, meaning that you are living in a state of continuous struggle, unhappiness, or stress in which no light appears at the end of the tunnel. Examples of continuous struggle include:

- Chronic illness (including untreated thyroid disease)
- Unhealthy relationships
- Poverty and/or economic worries
- Job stress

A third trigger for situational depression is an absence of resolution regarding past traumas and abuses you suffered as a child or younger adult.

In the absence of thyroid disease, one out of five people in North America suffer from at least one episode of depression in their lifetime. At least twice as many women suffer from depression as men.

Sadness Versus Depression

The million-dollar question is whether you are just sad or depressed. Everyone experiences sadness, bad days, and bad moods. Feeling sad is not the same thing as depression. Sadness is characterized by sad feelings, whereas the main feature of depression is numbness. The main thing to remember about sadness versus depression is that sadness lifts, while depression persists. Feelings of sadness and grief are definitely common and normal in an infinite variety of circumstances.

Symptoms of Unipolar Depression

It's impossible to define what a normal mood is, since we all have such complex personalities and exhibit different moods throughout a given week, or even a given day. But it's not impossible for you to define what a normal mood is for you. You know how you feel when you're functional: you're eating, sleeping, interacting with friends and family, and being productive, active, and generally interested in the daily goings-on in life. Depression is when you feel you've lost the ability to function for a prolonged period of time, or, even if you're functioning at a reasonable level as seen by the outside world, you've lost interest in participating in life.

The symptoms of unipolar depression vary from person to person but can include some or all of the following:

- Feelings of sadness and/or "empty" mood
- Difficulty sleeping (usually waking up frequently in the middle of the night)
- Loss of energy and feelings of fatigue and lethargy
- Change in appetite (usually a loss of appetite)
- Difficulty thinking, concentrating, or making decisions
- Loss of interest in formerly pleasurable activities, including sex

- Anxiety or panic attacks (this may also be a symptom of thyrotoxicosis, discussed in Chapter 3)
- Obsessing over negative experiences or thoughts
- Feeling guilty, worthless, hopeless, or helpless
- Feeling restless and irritable
- Thinking about death or suicide

Managing Unipolar Depression

When your depression is related to life events, talk therapy is the first logical step. Talk therapy can also be combined with antidepressant medications. Before you accept antidepressant medications, make sure to have a thyroid function test to detect for mild, moderate, or severe hypothyroidism. Many people who are diagnosed with depression and have mild hypothyroidism report improvement when they are treated with thyroid hormone. However, when you have a thyroid condition and depression independently of one another, the fact that your depression persists after your thyroid problem is treated does not necessarily mean your thyroid is acting up again.

Anxiety, Panic Disorder, and Thyroid Disease

Generalized anxiety disorder (GAD) and panic attacks are commonly confused with or aggravated by thyrotoxicosis. As previously outlined, when you're thyrotoxic, the number of beta-adrenergic receptors increase in your body's cells. This makes you much more sensitive to the effects of your own adrenaline and, even if you are ordinarily able to cope with various stressors, predisposes you to panic attacks and greater anxiety. The key to managing panic attacks and anxiety related to thyrotoxicosis is treatment with a beta-blocker (see Chapter 3).

Obviously, not everyone who suffers from anxiety and panic is thyrotoxic. You can be coping with other types of thyroid problems and become anxious from worrying about your thyroid condition. And, of course, you have a life outside of your thyroid condition. In the general population, other causes of anxiety are usually normal, garden-variety problems. Worrying about jobs, finances, relationships, and health are all common reasons for anxiety. But when you're under increased stress, normal worries can cross over into anxiety and low-level anxiety can also worsen.

Managing Anxiety and Panic

If you've ruled out thyrotoxicosis and do not require a beta-blocker, talk therapy (specifically, cognitive behavioral therapy) is an excellent way to manage anxiety and panic. This style of therapy can teach you to anticipate the situations and bodily sensations that are associated with panic attacks; having this awareness can help you control the attacks. There are also a number of mental exercises that can help you control hyperventilating or fearful thoughts that could heighten the panic in the throes of an attack. For instance, by replacing the thought "I'm going to faint" with "I'm just hyperventilating—I can handle this," panic attacks can be calmed before the "complete fear" takes over and the symptoms worsen.

Your doctor may also prescribe antidepressants or tranquilizers, depending on how severe your anxiety and panic are and whether they are affecting your ability to function normally.

Heart Disease and Thyroid Disease: A Troublesome Duo

Both untreated hypothyroidism (see Chapter 2) and thyrotoxicosis (see Chapter 3) can lead to cardiovascular complications (complications involving the heart, arteries, and veins) or a worsening of risk factors for cardiovascular disease. The term *heart disease* generally refers to any type of heart trouble, including irregular or rapid heart rhythms; blockages of the blood supply to the heart muscle causing chest pain (angina) or a heart attack (myocardial infarction); or weakening of the pumping of the heart, causing congestive heart failure. The term *atherosclerotic cardiovascular disease* (ASCVD) refers to fatty blockages of blood vessels anywhere in the body. When they occur in the coronary arteries that feed the heart muscle, they put you at risk for a heart attack. When ASCVD occurs in blood vessels in the

Chandra's Story: Nothing Gives Me Pleasure, Not Even Thyroid Hormone

I was diagnosed with Hashimoto's disease in my early forties, around the time that my mother was dying of pancreatic cancer. I was treated with thyroid hormone, but I still didn't feel right. I couldn't put my finger on it, exactly. It was as though I lost something. I was very active in my church and used to enjoy participating in the various activities we planned throughout the year, but I just lost interest. I stopped going, and I couldn't find anything I wanted to do anymore. I sort of just laid around like a lump all the time. I searched the Internet and found a lot of thyroid patients like me who said that they couldn't convert their thyroid hormone properly and that I was just feeling hypothyroid. My doctor told me that my TSH was normal and that my thyroid hormone levels were normal, too. He said that I might be depressed because of my mother's death and sent me to a grief counselor. The grief counselor thought I was depressed, and my doctor told me that there are lots of people with normal thyroid glands who are depressed, so why not me?

brain, they put you at risk for having a stroke, in which the part of the brain fed by the blocked blood vessel dies. When ASCVD affects arteries that feed your arms or your legs, it causes peripheral vascular disease. In addition, some people have heart disease that may not be related to ASCVD that affects the way the heart beats. Normally, the heart beats at a regular rhythm of between fifty and ninety beats per minute. Any disturbance of this rhythm is called an arrhythmia, and rapid rhythms are called tachyarrhythmias.

In thyroid patients who are otherwise healthy, these cardiovascular complications disappear or resolve as soon as you return to a euthyroid state, or normal thyroid function. In thyroid patients who have preexisting cardiovascular disease or who have risk factors for cardiovascular disease (obesity, smoking), untreated hypothyroidism or thyrotoxicosis can accelerate the worsening of cardiovascular problems. This section will briefly summarize the range of heart problems that can be complicated by thyroid disease.

Heart Complications from Hypothyroidism

Hypothyroidism slows down the heart, causing a slow pulse called bradycardia. This might cause decreased exercise tolerance, shortness of breath, or a feeling of being winded when you try to exert yourself. Prolonged hypothyroidism will also lead to the accumulation of fluids, called lymphedema, which can swell your hands and feet and mimic the type of edema seen with congestive heart failure. Because your arteries require thyroid hormone to relax, hypothyroidism causes them to tense up, resulting in high blood pressure. People with chronically weakened hearts from underlying ASCVD may not be able to pump blood very easily through these constricted blood vessels, worsening congestive heart failure with fluid accumulating in the lower limbs or in the lungs. Hypothyroid-induced edema can aggravate any existing congestive heart failure or might even be mistaken for congestive heart failure.

For most people with hypothyroidism, the most serious early complication is high blood pressure, which can increase the risk of a heart attack or stroke as well as congestive heart failure. Hypothyroidism also increases cholesterol levels, which can increase the development of blockages in arteries (atherosclerosis), likewise leading to increased risk of a heart attack or stroke as well as congestive heart failure. Sometimes people are misdiagnosed with congestive heart failure when hypothyroidism is the problem.

Congestive Heart Failure

The term *congestive heart failure* means that the heart is weakened and not pumping well. This is usually caused by long-standing problems such as damaged heart valves, high blood pressure, damage to the heart muscle, or, rarely, congenital heart defects—a variety of heart defects that could have been present at birth.

Heart failure usually develops over a period of years. When people with heart failure become hypothyroid, the heart weakens further and this condition can worsen. In addition, since the blood vessels throughout the body require thyroid hormone to relax, hypothyroidism makes it more difficult to push blood through them, a condition called increased peripheral vascular resistance. This makes it even more difficult for the left ventricle to pump blood forward and worsens the heart failure.

In people with normal thyroid function, the heart enhances its pumping action by beating faster. In hypothyroidism, the heart beats much slower and cannot compensate for heart failure by beating faster. It is very unusual for hypothyroidism, on its own, to weaken the heart sufficiently to cause heart failure. It's important to look for primary heart problems and treat them in addition to treating the hypothyroidism. If you have underlying heart failure that predated hypothyroidism or was unveiled as a result of hypothyroidism, treatment with lifestyle changes, blood pressure and cholesterol-lowering medications, or possibly surgery may be necessary.

Hypertension

About 10 to 20 percent of people with hypothyroidism suffer from hypertension, or high blood pressure, which can lead to heart failure if severe and left untreated for long periods of time. It can also lead to a heart attack or stroke. In the general population, target blood pressure readings are less than 140 over 80 ($-140/80$). Readings greater than 140/85 are considered too high, although readings of just under 144/88 are sometimes considered borderline in an otherwise healthy person. For the general population, 140/85 is "lecture time," when your doctor will begin to counsel you about dietary and lifestyle habits. By 150/90, many people are prescribed an antihypertensive drug, which is designed to lower blood pressure.

In the absence of thyroid disease, it's known that obesity, smoking, and a high-sodium diet can put you at risk for hypertension. Genetic factors are very important; your risks for hypertension are much higher if it runs in your family and certain ethnic groups have higher risks. High blood pressure can also be caused by kidney disorders, which are prevalent in people with diabetes, or by pregnancy. High blood pressure is treated in people with thyroid disease by a two-pronged approach, treating both problems—which may also involve lifestyle changes and antihypertensive medications. If your blood pressure returns to normal, you can discuss with your doctor whether you are able to come off of the medications.

High Cholesterol and Hypothyroidism

Hypothyroidism can increase cholesterol in people whose cholesterol levels would ordinarily be normal while euthyroid. If you have high cholesterol that predates your hypothyroidism, your already high cholesterol level can jump off the charts. High cholesterol is dangerous because the excess cholesterol in your blood can lead to narrowed arteries (ASCVD), which in turn can lead to a heart attack or stroke. In the absence of hypothyroidism, saturated fat is often a culprit when it comes to high cholesterol, but the highest levels of cholesterol are due to genetic features affecting the creation or disposal of cholesterol in the liver. Familial hypercholesterolemia refers to a genetic cause for high cholesterol that does not respond adequately to diet modification.

Hypothyroidism can increase the levels of LDL-cholesterol in the blood (the so-called "bad" cholesterol). The liver is the organ responsible for ridding the body of cholesterol as well as making it. Much of hypothyroidism's effect is caused by increasing the absorption of cholesterol from bile (a substance made by the liver), preventing the usual loss of the body's own cholesterol in the intestines. In addition, the hypothyroid liver seems unable to effectively clear this cholesterol, contributing to its increased levels. A few months after starting the appropriate dosage of levothyroxine, sufficient to make your TSH level normal, the elevating effects of hypothyroidism on cholesterol levels should be gone. Of course, if you have underlying elevated cholesterol levels, you may still need to treat your high cholesterol by modifying your diet and taking cholesterol-lowering medications.

Heart Complications from Thyrotoxicosis

Even when people feel few other symptoms of thyrotoxicosis, they usually feel the heart symptoms. Thyrotoxicosis, as explained in

Chapter 3, speeds up the heart rate by increasing the sensitivity of the heart to catecholamines (adrenaline and related hormones). In otherwise healthy people, this can lead to palpitations and tachycardia (fast pulse). In people with underlying cardiovascular disease or risk factors for cardiovascular disease, thyrotoxicosis can lead to atrial fibrillation and arrhythmias (abnormal heart rhythms). The stress placed on the heart can aggravate angina (chest pain) as well as a type of congestive heart failure called high-output congestive heart failure.

Palpitations and Racing Heart

The classic heart complications associated with thyrotoxicosis are a very fast pulse and heart palpitations. If you are hyperthyroid as a result of Graves' disease (see Chapter 3), once your thyroid hormone levels are reduced to normal, these symptoms will disappear. Treatment with either antithyroid medication or beta-blockers (see Chapter 3) can slow the heartbeat and prevent the consequences of a racing heart, such as heart failure or atrial fibrillation. Once thyroid function is restored to normal, you can usually stop taking beta-blockers.

Complications with Amiodarone

Amiodarone is a potent medicine used to treat heart rhythm disturbances. It is infamous for causing three different types of thyroid problems. This is partly because the amiodarone drug contains a large amount of iodine and partly because the amiodarone tends to stay inside the body for many months, even though you may stop taking it. It is also because some people have a reaction to the amiodarone in which it causes an inflammation of the thyroid gland, releasing stored thyroid hormones. If you're taking this drug, make sure your doctor checks your thyroid function.

Chest Pain (Angina)

Chest pain or discomfort due to coronary heart disease is called angina. People with underlying heart disease may have worsening of angina when they are thyrotoxic. The heart's metabolism is increased by the excess thyroid hormone, increasing the oxygen and sugar demands of the muscle. The acceleration of the heart rate also places additional demands on the heart muscle. Partially blocked coronary arteries are unable to meet this increased demand for heart-feeding blood. The chest pain of angina (angina pectoris) is the sign that there is not enough blood feeding the heart. If left untreated, this condition can develop into a heart attack, in which part of the heart muscle dies, putting the person at risk of death if it is severe enough. Treatment consists of efforts to reduce the stress and demands put on the heart by using beta-blockers and to enhance the blood flow through the coronary arteries either by using drugs that expand their diameter or with a balloon catheter to reduce blockages.

Fatigue: Sleep Disorder or Thyroid Disease?

The symptoms of hypothyroidism (see Chapter 2), together with the symptoms of thyrotoxicosis (see Chapter 3) can exacerbate the normal fatigue that is a part of your daily life. However, these symptoms may also mask a sleep disorder, now the most commonly diagnosed cause of fatigue and sleep deprivation.

Be Informed: Misinformation About Fatigue and Hypothyroidism

A lot of patients treated for hypothyroidism claim they feel tired and, therefore, must still be hypothyroid. This has led to bizarre explanations about how TSH works and to the T4/T3 conversion myth (see Chapter 1). Unfortunately, fatigue is a factor for just about everyone these days, and the most common cause of fatigue is one of the many types of sleep disorders. If you ask 100 people with healthy thyroid glands if they suffer from fatigue, more than half will raise their hands. Fatigue is *not* a symptom of your thyroid disorder if you have a normal TSH level and normal free T4 levels. Some patients insist that persistent fatigue combined with normal TSH levels means that their thyroid hormone must not be working or that they are not converting T3 into T4, but this cannot be true if their TSH is normal. As explained in Chapter 1, the T4/T3 conversion problem theory is false.

Normal Fatigue

Lifestyle factors are largely responsible for most people's fatigue. When hypothyroidism is added to normal fatigue, however, it can be overwhelming. In these cases, the lifestyle changes that can remedy normal fatigue can help you feel less fatigued while going through a bout of untreated hypothyroidism. Whether you're euthyroid, hypo-thyroid, or thyrotoxic, for better sleep try the following tips.

- Regular bedtime hours. Go to bed at the same time every night.
- Regular wake-up hour. Try to wake up around the same time every morning.
- Daily sun exposure. Exposure to natural outdoor light during the day helps with sleep.
- A cool, dark, and quiet room at bedtime. Lower the temperature at night or open a window. Use earplugs if necessary, and pull down shades or draw curtains.

There are two times during a twenty-four-hour period when we are most inclined to feel sleepy regardless of how much sleep we've had. The first period is between about midnight and 7:00 A.M., when most of us do sleep. But the second period is after lunch, which in many cultures is siesta or nap time, between 1:00 and 3:00 P.M. If you're getting less sleep at night, taking a nap between 1:00 and 3:00 P.M. can help to combat fatigue in people with more flexible hours, or in people who work night shifts.

If you're getting regular sleep and are euthyroid but find you're dosing off during the day or still feel tired, this could be a sign of a sleep disorder. A range of sleep disorders can contribute to normal fatigue. Some sleep disorders, such as sleep apnea (discussed later in this chapter), can even point to an unrecognized thyroid problem, as the apnea can be caused by a goiter or even a large nodule that may be obstructing breathing at night.

Sleep Deprivation

Sleep deprivation refers to being deprived of the recommended hours of sleep for healthy adults. Sleep deprivation can dramatically worsen fatigue in people who are hypothyroid. In people who are thyrotoxic, sleep deprivation can contribute to exhaustion, but sleep is difficult anyway because the body is "racing" at night, which interferes with a good night's sleep.

There are two phases of sleep: rapid eye movement (REM) and nonrapid eye movement. REM sleep is when we dream, an important component of mental health. REM sleep is also our deepest sleep, which is when, researchers believe, various hormones are reset and energy stores are replenished. Sleep is therefore an active state that affects our physical and mental well-being. Insufficient restful sleep can result in mental and physical health problems.

There is a misconception that as we get older, we need less sleep. This is not so; we need just as much as sleep as always, but we often get less sleep. What happens is that our ability to achieve quality sleep for long periods of time diminishes as we age. The older we get, the more fragile our sleep becomes, and thus it can be more easily disturbed by light, noise, and pain (such as arthritis). It's common for various medical conditions to interfere with sleep; in the case of thyroid disease, this is usually the restlessness, anxiety, and racing heart of thyrotoxicosis (see Chapter 3).

Sleep Disorders

Sleep disorders are far more common in the general population than hypothyroidism. Many hypothyroid patients, when diagnosed and treated for a sleep disorder, begin to feel better again. The following is a brief overview of common sleep disorders. Sometimes sleep apnea can be diagnosed when a goiter or thyroid tumor is the cause.

Sleep Apnea

Sleep apnea (*apnea* means "want of breath" in Greek) is a breathing disorder in which breathing interruptions during sleep awaken you. One type of apnea is central and the other type is obstructive. Central sleep apnea occurs when the brain fails to send the appropriate signals to the breathing muscles that cause you to breathe in and out. More common, however, is obstructive sleep apnea. This occurs when air cannot flow in or out of your nose or mouth. This can be linked to a growth or tumor in the neck or throat area, such as a goiter or a large thyroid nodule. In other people, apnea is the result of throat and tongue muscles relaxing during sleep, which can partially block airways. Obesity can also lead to apnea, as an excess amount of tissue can narrow breathing airways. Signs that you may have sleep apnea are persistent loud snoring at night and daytime sleepiness. Frequent long pauses in breathing during sleep followed by choking and gasping for breath is an obvious sign of sleep apnea. Some people may find they wake up frequently due to the brain forcing an arousal each time they stop breathing. Ultimately, this leads to daytime fatigue due to lack of sleep. Far more serious problems are also linked to sleep apnea, including higher rates of hypertension, heart disease, heart attack, and stroke. If you think you have sleep apnea, a pulmonary specialist (a doctor who specializes in lungs and breathing) can treat it with various methods.

Insomnia

Insomnia causes poor quality sleep because you cannot fall asleep, you wake up a lot during the night and cannot fall back asleep (also a sign of depression), you wake up too early in the morning, or you have the sense that your sleep is fitful or unrefreshing. Most causes of insomnia are linked to mental or emotional stress, and it is seen more frequently in people over age sixty, in women, and in people who suffer from depression.

Restless Legs Syndrome (RLS)

Restless legs syndrome is a sleep disorder characterized by tingling sensations in the legs or arms while sitting or lying down. The sensations are described as creeping, crawling, tingling, pulling, or painful. In many cases the sensations interfere with your ability to fall asleep or to stay asleep.

Burnout or Hypothyroidism?

Burnout is now a common term in all health-care literature and is characterized by physical and emotional exhaustion, feeling personally disconnected with one's friends and family, and feeling nonproductive. Signs of burnout include low morale, exhaustion, poor concentration, and feelings of helplessness and depression, as well as physical problems such as bowel problems, poor appetite, cramps, and headaches. Bouts of untreated hypothyroidism or thyrotoxicosis can dramatically magnify burnout.

Menopause and Thyroid Disease

When it comes to menopause, women with thyroid disease have a little more to be concerned about than women without thyroid disease. All postmenopausal women are at an increased risk of heart disease, which is the leading cause of death for postmenopausal women. But in postmenopausal women with untreated hypothyroidism, hyperthyroidism, or thyrotoxicosis, cardiovascular changes can damage the heart, magnifying the normal risk of heart disease that exists in the general female population. In addition, hyperthyroidism or thyrotoxicosis can speed the process of osteoporosis, which is also a risk for women after menopause.

In women who had normal thyroid function prior to menopause, the signs of thyroid disease can be masked by perimenopausal symptoms. This means that thyroid disease can be missed, aggravating menopausal and postmenopausal risks of other diseases, such as osteoporosis or heart disease. Women might also be mistakenly told they are perimenopausal when they are not. It's important to note that the incidence of mild hypothyroidism or subclinical hypothyroidism steadily rises with age, increasing from 10 percent in the premenopausal age group to 20 percent in the postmenopausal age group. When you notice signs of perimenopause (changing periods, hot flashes, trouble sleeping, etc.), make sure to request a thyroid function test to rule out thyroid disease as the cause of symptoms (e.g., thyrotoxicosis or hyperthyroidism) or to see if you need to alter your current thyroid hormone dosage.

Thyroid Disease and Osteoporosis

Postmenopausal women have the highest risk of developing osteoporosis (bone loss) as a result of estrogen loss, and osteoporosis can be aggravated by thyrotoxicosis. Osteoporosis increases your risk of bone fractures; fully 70 percent of all hip fractures are a direct result of osteoporosis. Maintaining bone mass and good bone health is your best defense against osteoporosis.

Be Informed:
Beware of Bioidentical Hormones

If you are considering taking hormone replacement therapy (HRT) for menopausal symptoms, beware of bioidentical hormones; the FDA has determined that this is a marketing term and is not medically meaningful. Bioidentical hormones are unregulated, and many unskilled and unlicensed practitioners are prescribing them, falsely claiming that they protect against breast cancer. They are usually sold by compounding pharmacies as a "natural" form of HRT synthesized from plants, but they frequently contain other hormones, including T3, which can be dangerous if you are already taking thyroid hormone. The truth is, all forms of estrogen and progesterone carry the same risks and benefits. Aim for something that is FDA-approved and regulated, which your doctor can discuss with you.

One of the most common questions that women taking thyroid hormone ask is: What is the link between thyroid disease and osteoporosis? Contrary to what some women think, the link has nothing to do with calcitonin, which the thyroid also produces (discussed in Chapter 1).

Thyroid hormone will speed up or slow down bone cells just as it speeds or slows other processes in our bodies, such as our metabolism. Osteoblasts are the cells responsible for building bone, while osteoclasts are cells that remove old bone so that it can be replaced by new bone. When you are thyrotoxic, osteoclasts get overstimulated; in short, they go nuts. They begin to remove bone faster than it can be replaced by the osteoblasts, which are not affected by too much thyroid hormone. The result is too much bone removal and subsequent bone loss.

Women who have had a thyroidectomy to treat thyroid cancer need to be on a slightly higher dosage of thyroid hormone to suppress all thyroid-stimulating hormone activity. Thus, they may live in a state of mild thyrotoxicosis. Postmenopausal women on thyroid hormone should have their levels checked every year to adjust their dosage accordingly.

Thyroid Disease After Sixty

Roughly 4 to 7 percent of people over age sixty are definitely hypothyroid. It's also suspected that a much greater percentage of people over sixty have subclinical hypothyroidism that frequently goes unrecognized and untreated. Meanwhile, less than 1 percent of people over sixty suffer from hyperthyroidism. In either case, the symptoms of hypothyroidism and hyperthyroidism are different in older people and do not manifest in the same ways as in a younger person. It is recommended that everyone over sixty be screened for hypothyroidism annually with a TSH test. Older thyroid patients report that they feel better once treated with thyroid hormone and that a lot of their vague health problems get better or even disappear.

Hypothyroidism After Sixty

Most causes of primary hypothyroidism in people over sixty are due to Hashimoto's thyroiditis (see Chapter 2). Hashimoto's disease in younger people frequently causes an enlarged thyroid or goiter. In those over sixty, Hashimoto's disease tends to quietly damage the thyroid gland until it shrivels up. These people could walk around for years with unrecognized Hashimoto's disease unless a thyroid function test was done. Unlike younger people with Hashimoto's disease, thyroid antibody testing in older people is very unreliable as well; many older people with these antibodies are not hypothyroid.

Hypothyroidism in people over age sixty can increase cholesterol levels, which can in turn exacerbate heart disease. Hypothyroidism can also worsen depression, cognitive function, arthritis and muscular aches, memory, respiratory problems, and sleep apnea. It can also aggravate preexisting dementia.

Treating Hypothyroidism in Persons over Sixty

In people over age sixty with a TSH of greater than 10, there is a clear benefit to treatment with thyroid hormone. In people with a TSH of 5–10, treatment is also likely to be helpful, although the benefits in symptom relief are much less obvious. The risk of thyrotoxicosis from excessive dosages of thyroid hormone in an older person with either heart problems and/or osteoporosis means that thyroid hormone dosing needs to follow a "start low, go very slow" approach. Experienced endocrinologists are often able to better choose appropriate dosages that are not excessive without having to delay treatment by starting too low. People over sixty also require less thyroid hormone than younger people, which is why starting doses of thyroid hormone are advised to be conservative. It is in this group, especially, where T3 in combination with T4 (see Chapter 10) has not been properly studied and could have harmful effects. Similarly, "natural" thyroid hormone or thyroid extract is not recommended for this group.

A Note on Heart Disease

In people over age sixty, hypothyroidism symptoms can obscure heart diseases such as angina. Also, less commonly, swelling from hypothyroidism may be mistaken for congestive heart failure. In addition, people in heart failure have a faster pulse than normal; the hypothyroid heart is slower than normal, usually less than 60 beats per minute. There are other distinctions between hypothyroidism and congestive heart failure, but those truly in congestive heart failure don't usually have other hypothyroid symptoms at the same time.

Mischa's Story: Hypothyroidism, not Heart Disease

My eighty-five-year-old mother was complaining of swollen arms and legs, and we were told by her primary care doctor that she had severe edema from heart failure. Then we were sent to a cardiologist, who told us this wasn't true. After doing some tests, the cardiologist discovered she was severely hypothyroid and put her on thyroid hormone. She got better in a couple of weeks. I always wonder what would have happened to her if her hypothyroidism wasn't caught? And how many older women like her are told they have heart failure and not hypothyroidism?

Thyrotoxicosis in Persons over Sixty

Hyperthyroidism from Graves' disease (see Chapter 3) or a nodule (see Chapter 5) occurs in less than 1 percent of the population over age sixty. In fact, it is less than one-tenth as common as hypothyroidism in the same population. When it does occur, the symptoms are not obvious and do not clearly indicate the diagnosis of Graves' disease to the doctor in the same way as in a younger person. Similar to hypothyroidism, hyperthyroidism can be insidious in the over-sixty crowd; it can manifest as "apathetic" hyperthyroidism. This means that many of the symptoms in young people are absent in the older population, and thyroid disease may contribute to failing health, but may not be obvious or easy to spot. This is one reason why screening for subclinical thyroid disease in older groups of people is recommended.

The Autoimmune Disease Collection Package

If you have one autoimmune disease, you are more likely to start a "collection" of them. This is especially true if you're a woman, since women are more prone to autoimmune diseases than men. Stress has been observed to be a definite trigger for autoimmune disorders, but no one really understands how this works and why this is. Pregnancy is a major factor in autoimmune disease; women are most prone to developing autoimmune diseases in their first trimester and in the first six months after delivery (postpartum).

Autoimmune thyroid diseases are associated with other conditions, particularly a condition known as myasthenia gravis. Some people with Hashimoto's thyroiditis or Graves' disease may also have one or more of the following: anemia, rheumatoid arthritis, lupus, Type 1 diabetes (not to be confused with Type 2 diabetes, which is not autoimmune), and Addison's disease. The basic rule is that if you have one autoimmune disease, you should be alert to the early signs and symptoms of other autoimmune diseases.

8

Thyroid Disease and New Life

Fertility, Pregnancy, Postpartum, and Neonatal Issues

THIS CHAPTER DISCUSSES issues for distinct groups of women and mothers: women trying to get pregnant; pregnant women with unrecognized or subclinical thyroid disease; pregnant women with preexisting thyroid disease; women who first discover or develop a thyroid problem during pregnancy; women who first discover or develop a thyroid problem within the first six months of delivery; and finally, thyroid disease in newborns and infants.

It's important to remember that autoimmune thyroid diseases, such as Hashimoto's thyroiditis (see Chapter 2) or Graves' disease (see Chapter 3), frequently strike during the first trimester of a pregnancy or within the first six months after delivery. That said, you should note that preexisting autoimmune thyroid disease as well as other autoimmune diseases tend to improve during a pregnancy but can worsen after delivery. Thyroid nodules and thyroid cancer can also be first discovered during a pregnancy; see chapters 5 and 6 for more information.

One of the aims of this chapter is to educate you about the potential dangers of untreated thyroid disease during pregnancy to both the mother and fetus. All women planning pregnancy and their prenatal health-care team should be aware of the following facts discussed in this chapter:

- Pregnant women with hypothyroidism (overt or subclinical) are at an increased risk for premature delivery.
- Pregnant women who have antibodies for autoimmune thyroid disease are at an increased risk for miscarriage, postpartum thyroiditis, Graves' disease, and hypothyroidism.
- Children born to mothers with hypothyroidism or high thyroid-stimulating hormone levels are at a higher risk of intellectual or motor impairment.

Thyroid Disease and Fertility

Approximately 6.1 million couples experience infertility each year, according to the American Society for Reproductive Medicine (ASRM). Surveys indicate about 15 percent of all couples will experience infertility at some time during their reproductive lives. When there are identifiable causes for infertility, it's split evenly between male-factor and female-factor infertility. Roughly 20 percent of the time, the cause is unknown. The most common cause of infertility, however, is age. Table 8.1 indicates rates of fecundity (the ability to produce offspring) according to age. Age-related fecundity may be blamed when a thyroid disorder is actually the cause.

Table 8.1 Fertility Through the Ages

Age	Likelihood of getting pregnant*	Likelihood of infertility
20–24	100%	3%
25–29	94%	5%
30–34	86%	8%
35–39	70%	15%
40–44	36%	32%
45–49	5%	69%
50+	0%	100%

*Presuming optimum health
Source: Adapted from Khatamee, Masood, M.D. "Infertility: A Preventable Epidemic?" *International Journal of Fertility* 33, no. 4 (1988): 246–51.

Karla's Story: A Five-Year Delay

I got pregnant later than I had hoped—at forty-one. When I started trying at thirty-six, I was warned that my age would be a problem, and when I didn't get pregnant and my cycles were irregular, I was told to start thinking about IVF (in vitro fertilization). We didn't want to go through fertility treatments; I knew a lot of women who had bad experiences with the fertility drugs. I switched insurance plans and needed to see a different primary care doctor, and she asked me, "Has anyone checked your thyroid levels recently?" I was apparently hypothyroid (my TSH was 25). I didn't feel anything except a little tired, but who isn't tired? I was put on levothyroxine, and I got pregnant pretty quickly after that. I was frustrated that a small thing like this may have wasted five good years of trying.

If you're planning a pregnancy, start with a thyroid test to make sure that any problems with your cycles are not related to either hypothyroidism or hyperthyroidism. In addition, unrecognized thyroid disease can lead to miscarriage or fetal development problems. If your thyroid tests are normal prior to conception, you can rule out thyroid disease as a cause of infertility; if thyroid disease is discovered, you can restore fertility by treating it. If your thyroid is normal at conception, you should repeat TSH tests and thyroid antibody tests on the discovery of the pregnancy and have them checked monthly during your routine prenatal exams if the thyroid antibody tests are positive. Although not yet common practice, it's reasonable that TSH tests be done at regular intervals on all fertile women (regardless of plans for pregnancy), because they could become pregnant and may not seek medical care until well into their pregnancy if they do have a thyroid problem.

If You Have Had Radioactive Iodine Therapy

If you were treated for hyperthyroidism or thyroid cancer with radioactive iodine, you should plan not to get pregnant for about six months afterward, although there isn't any definite evidence that pregnancy prior to this waiting period after RAI is harmful. There is one exception, which has more to do with hypothyroidism: if you were treated for thyroid cancer and were made hypothyroid for a treatment or a scan, you must wait until your thyroid hormone levels are normal before you try to conceive. Hypothyroidism in the early stages of fetal development can be harmful to the fetus. Otherwise, pregnancies should proceed normally as long as you're taking sufficient doses of your thyroid hormone replacement and your TSH level is monitored monthly; doses frequently need to be adjusted during pregnancy.

Normal Pregnancy Discomforts: How They Relate to Thyroid Disease

Common discomforts of pregnancy may mimic or mask hypothyroidism, which is why regular TSH testing is encouraged. If you are vomiting because of morning sickness, however, you may not be ingesting adequate amounts of iodine. The recommended total daily iodine intake should be 220 mcg per day for pregnant women and 290 mcg per day for lactating women. Dairy products are very high in iodine content, so if you're meeting your calcium requirements, you're probably fine. The iodine in milk varies greatly (depending upon the season, the cow's feed, and the location), averaging around 250 mcg per liter (60 mcg per cup). Prenatal vitamins, which most North American pregnant women take, contain at least 150 mcg of iodine per daily dose. If you take these vitamins with a glass of milk, you should be fine. If you're unable to keep any liquids down, your physician should pay careful attention to *all* your nutritional needs, including iodine, to prevent malnutrition.

If you are suffering from severe morning sickness in early pregnancy, this may be a sign of gestational thyrotoxicosis, a transient form of thyrotoxicosis. It's believed that morning sickness can become increasingly severe because of the overproduction of thyroid hormone.

Morning Sickness and Thyroid Hormone Replacement

Morning sickness also presents other problems for women who take thyroid replacement hormone (for preexisting or newly diagnosed thyroid diseases). Morning sickness may be mild, moderate, or severe. For more severe cases, the nausea and vomiting begins between six and eight weeks after your last menstrual period, persists strongly until about fourteen weeks after your last menstrual period, and then either disappears or gets much better. But it can persist well into the second trimester too and can even last the duration of the pregnancy.

If you are taking thyroxine, the problem with nonstop nausea and vomiting is that your thyroid hormone pill could be poorly absorbed, leaving you hypothyroid, which is dangerous to fetal health. If you are in doubt about whether your thyroid hormone pill came out with your breakfast, it's probably all right to take an additional tablet as long as this isn't too frequent an event. In extreme situations, your physician could give you your thyroxine medication as an injection into your muscle or under your skin.

Pregnancy and Preexisting Thyroid Disease

If you are hypothyroid or are taking thyroid hormone replacement for a thyroid condition diagnosed prior to your current pregnancy, it's important to have your thyroid levels assessed monthly. Your target TSH level should be between 0.5 and 3 so that your dosages of thyroid hormone replacement can be appropriately adjusted, which is necessary for the growing fetus. Total T4 assessments are useless, since T4 naturally rises because of increased thyroxine-binding globulin (TBG); this is due to increased levels of estrogen during pregnancy. Although very little thyroid hormone will cross over from you to the baby, the little that does is very important, since normal thyroid hormone levels in you are critical for proper fetal development until your baby develops his or her own thyroid gland. Sometimes a change in dosage is needed because requirements for thyroid hormone can increase during pregnancy. It's normal to require as much as a 30 to 50 percent increase in your dosage. Your doctor should monitor your TSH level and increase your dosage as necessary. Since prenatal vitamins often contain iron, it's important to take them at night so that the iron doesn't interfere with the absorption of your morning thyroid pill.

Pregnancy and Graves' Disease

Taking antithyroid medication (see Chapter 3) for Graves' disease while pregnant is perfectly safe, and you should continue this medication so long as you're under the supervision of a doctor. In fact, taking this medication may protect the baby in your womb from the effects of thyroid-stimulating antibody, which crosses from you into the baby's circulation. The dosage of the antithyroid medication usually needs to be decreased during pregnancy for two reasons. First, your baby's thyroid is more sensitive to these drugs than your own, and, second, Graves' disease activity changes during the course of your pregnancy.

If you're pregnant with active Graves' disease that was newly discovered, you must start antithyroid drugs as soon as possible. You should remain slightly hyperthyroid so the baby's thyroid antibodies can be properly suppressed.

If you are pregnant and have a history of previously treated Graves' disease, there is still a risk that you could have a hyperthyroid baby because you may still be making thyroid-stimulating immunoglobulin (TSI). Without a working thyroid, you'll never know, but TSI could still cross the placenta into the baby. In the case of previously treated Graves' disease, you should request that your prenatal health care provider monitor the fetal heart rate during the pregnancy to look for signs that suggest fetal thyrotoxicosis; under rare circumstances, your health care provider may need a blood sample from the placenta to check thyroid hormone levels. If you've had a remission of Graves' disease, fetal thyrotoxicosis should not be a risk.

Gestational Thyroid Disease

For the most part, the causes of thyroid disease during pregnancy are the same as in the general population. And the most common thyroid diseases in pregnancy mirror the most common thyroid diseases in the general population: Hashimoto's disease (see Chapter 2) is the most common thyroid disease in pregnancy, followed by Graves' disease (see Chapter 3). In both cases, the risk spikes during the first three months of pregnancy, and then spikes again in the first six months

Rosita's Story: My Starry-Eyed Pregnancy

I was treated with radioactive iodine for my Graves' disease three years before I got pregnant, and so my thyroid was destroyed and I was taking thyroid hormone. Around my eleventh week, I noticed that my eyes started bulging and were bothering me. My doctor was at Brigham and Women's in Boston, and when he saw my eyes, he explained that even though I had no thyroid and was not hyperthyroid anymore, my Graves' disease was active, and that my thyroid antibodies were going to affect the baby unless I went on antithyroid medication. He explained that the baby's thyroid gland would be fully developed soon and that once that happened, the same antibodies that attacked my eyes would attack my baby's thyroid gland. So I went on the antithyroid medications for the remainder of my pregnancy, and the baby was okay but would have been really sick if I didn't take these drugs.

after delivery. Up to 20 percent of all women, particularly those with thyroid antibodies or insulin-dependent diabetes, will develop postpartum thyroiditis. This usually resolves on its own, but 25 percent of the time, it can leave women permanently hypothyroid.

Just as in the general population, pregnant women can develop hypothyroidism or thyrotoxicosis for other reasons, discussed in Chapters 2 and 3. What seems clear to thyroid researchers, however, is that pregnancy increases thyroid hormone requirements; increases the risks of iodine deficiency, which can increase the severity of preexisting hypothyroidism; can worsen preexisting Hashimoto's or Graves' disease; and can unveil overt hypothyroidism in women who had subclinical hypothyroidism prior to pregnancy.

Gestational Hypothyroidism

If hypothyroidism is suspected while you're pregnant, your doctor will give you a TSH test. Just as in nonpregnant women, your TSH levels will be increased if you're hypothyroid and you'll be treated with thyroid hormone replacement. Sometimes pregnancy itself can mask hypothyroid symptoms. For example, constipation, puffiness, and fatigue are all traits of pregnancy as well as of hypothyroidism. These symptoms will likely persist after delivery if your hypothyroidism remains untreated, and they can cause serious pregnancy complications and interfere with your postpartum health.

Gestational hypertension, preeclampsia, and eclampsia are more common in women with overt or subclinical hypothyroidism. These pregnancy complications may warrant early delivery or lead to premature delivery.

Gestational Thyrotoxicosis

Gestational thyrotoxicosis refers to a transient form of thyrotoxicosis caused by rising levels of human chorionic gonadotropin (HCG), which stimulate the thyroid gland to make thyroid hormone. This is usually found in women with severe morning sickness and is typically diagnosed toward the end of the first trimester. Gestational thyrotoxicosis usually resolves on its own after pregnancy. Temporary treatment with propranolol, a beta-blocker (see Chapter 3), may be used. However, the necessity of the beta-blocker and the length of time you're on one during pregnancy needs to be carefully monitored on a case-by-case basis by your doctor. If the thyrotoxicosis is very severe, antithyroid drugs, such as propylthiouracil (PTU), may be used in smaller than usual dosages.

Thyrotoxicosis Due to Molar Pregnancy

Roughly one in every fifteen hundred to two thousand pregnancies in North America will develop into a molar pregnancy, also known as a hydatidiform mole, a form of gestational trophoblastic neoplasia. Here the placenta, in a cruel and bizarre twist of biology, becomes precancerous. This condition is most frequently reported in Asian women and in women in the South Pacific and Mexico. One sign of a molar pregnancy is thyrotoxicosis, due to very high levels of HCG, which drop only slightly over time after the pregnancy ends. This is very rare, but molar pregnancy should be ruled out if you become thyrotoxic.

Gestational Hyperthyroidism

Diagnosis and treatment of hyperthyroidism during pregnancy presents some unique fetal and maternal considerations. First, the risk of miscarriage and stillbirth is increased if hyperthyroidism goes untreated. Second, the overall risks to you and the baby increase if the disease persists or is first recognized late in pregnancy. As in non-pregnant women, specific hyperthyroid symptoms usually indicate a problem, but here again, some of the classic symptoms, such as heat intolerance or palpitations, can mirror classic pregnancy complaints. Usually, symptoms such as bulgy eyes or a pronounced goiter give Graves' disease away. But because radioactive iodine scans or treatment are never performed during pregnancy, gestational hyperthyroidism can only be confirmed through a blood test. (If you are exposed to radioactive iodine during pregnancy because the pregnancy was not suspected, you may want to discuss the risks and the possibility of a therapeutic abortion with your practitioner.) If you are of an age to be fertile, you should get a pregnancy test before receiving any radioactive substance, either for scans or for treatments.

The treatment for hyperthyroidism in pregnancy is antithyroid medication. Propylthiouracil (PTU) or methimazole are most commonly used, but PTU is the one usually used during pregnancy (see Chapter 3). PTU, by suppressing the fetal thyroid, actually benefits the fetus. Since the fetal thyroid is slightly more sensitive to PTU than the mother's thyroid, the dose is slightly less than would completely normalize the mother's thyroid hormone levels.

Sometimes women discover they are allergic to PTU. If this happens, methimazole is used instead. When there is a problem with both drugs, sometimes a thyroidectomy during the second trimester is performed, although this is rare. In general, surgery is avoided during pregnancy because it can trigger a miscarriage.

Many times, hyperthyroidism becomes milder as the pregnancy progresses. When this happens, antithyroid medication can be tapered off slowly as the pregnancy reaches full term; often, normal thyroid function resumes after delivery. Careful thought should be given to breast-feeding, since radioactive iodine treatments should not be given while breastfeeding nor for at least one month after weaning (see page 144).

Sometimes beta-blockers such as propranolol are given in addition to PTU. However, this is something your physician must assess on a case-by-case basis because it is not usual care. It can be continued safely during pregnancy if absolutely necessary. One potential risk of using it for too long is having a smaller than average baby.

The Risk of Miscarriage

Studies indicate that women with antithyroid antibodies or with sub-clinical Hashimoto's disease or Graves' disease have a 32 percent risk of miscarriage, compared to a 16 percent risk in women without these conditions. The risk of miscarriage also rises due to age. In the general population of healthy pregnant women under age thirty-five, one in six pregnancies ends in miscarriage, with risk at its highest point during the first trimester.

Discovering Thyroid Nodules During Pregnancy

If you discover a nodule on your thyroid gland during pregnancy, investigation and treatment will vary depending on how far along you are in your pregnancy.

A fine needle aspiration biopsy (see Chapter 5) should be done to determine whether the nodule is benign or malignant (cancer). If it is malignant, surgery will probably be performed during the second trimester, which is considered the safest time for surgery. If a cancerous nodule is confirmed in the second trimester, surgery may still be performed if there is time. Otherwise, you might simply have to wait until after you deliver. If, however, a cancerous nodule is only first discovered well into the second trimester or in the third trimester, surgical treatment can usually wait until you deliver. Then you will be able to have the appropriate thyroid surgery, as discussed in Chapter 6.

After the Baby Is Born

During pregnancy your immune system is naturally suppressed to prevent your body from rejecting the fetus. After pregnancy, your immune system turns on again. This has a rebound effect; the immune system is so alert that it is almost too powerful and can develop auto-antibodies that attack normal tissue. This is what's known as an autoimmune disorder and may be one reason why women are more prone to thyroid autoimmune disorders after pregnancy. This scenario is like having a guard dog tied up for nine months and then let out—the dog will be feistier and may even attack its owner.

If you first develop an autoimmune thyroid disease, such as Graves' disease or Hashimoto's thyroiditis, after you deliver, you would undergo normal treatment for either disease, as outlined in Chapters 2 and 3. If you develop Graves' disease after delivery and are breastfeeding, you may continue breastfeeding while taking antithyroid medication, but you must not breastfeed if you're having radioactive iodine therapy or scans.

If you developed Graves' disease during pregnancy, the condition can get worse after delivery unless antithyroid drugs are continued.

If you were diagnosed and successfully treated for Graves' disease prior to pregnancy, you can sometimes suffer a relapse after delivery. Depending on its severity, some women can opt to postpone treatment until they're finished breastfeeding.

Postpartum Thyroiditis

Postpartum thyroiditis means "inflammation of the thyroid gland after delivery" and is often the culprit behind the so-called postpartum blues. Postpartum thyroiditis usually lasts six to nine months before it resolves on its own.

Postpartum thyroiditis is a general label referring to silent thyroiditis (see Chapter 4) occurring after delivery and causing mild thyrotoxicosis and/or a short-lived Hashimoto's-type of thyroiditis, resulting in mild hypothyroidism. Until quite recently, the mild hypothyroid and thyrotoxic symptoms were attributed simply to symptoms of postpartum depression or to those notorious maternal blues thought to be caused by the dramatic hormonal changes women experience after pregnancy. Recent studies, however, indicate that as many as 18 percent of all pregnant women experience transient thyroid problems and subsequent mild forms of thyrotoxicosis, hyperthyroidism, or hypothyroidism. This statistic does not account for the many women who develop Graves' disease either during or after pregnancy.

Generally, the silent thyroiditis or short-lived Hashimoto's thyroiditis lasts for only a few weeks. Often, women don't even realize what's wrong with them, because the symptoms are mild and usually associated with the natural fatigue that accompanies taking care of a newborn.

These conditions usually clear up by themselves. Short-lived Hashimoto's thyroiditis is usually more common than silent thyroiditis after delivery (although the difference is not significant), and, in more severe cases, thyroid hormone is administered temporarily to alleviate the hypothyroid symptoms.

If you have severe thyrotoxic symptoms, you may be placed on beta-blockers until the excess thyroid hormone is depleted. Regardless of whether you are given thyroid hormone or beta-blockers, you can usually still breastfeed safely. Women who experience this sudden thyroid flare-up tend to experience it with each subsequent pregnancy. Obviously, women who do experience postpartum thyroiditis are predisposed to thyroid disorders and seem to be vulnerable in that particular area.

Today, it should be standard practice for all pregnant women to have thyroid function tests after delivery. If your thyroid test is normal yet you still have symptoms of postpartum depression or maternal blues, then you can rule out an underlying thyroid problem.

Postpartum Thyroiditis, Blues, or Postpartum Depression?

If you look at the symptoms of hypothyroidism in Chapter 2, it's easy to see how they can be confused with the symptoms of postpartum depression, which affect as many as 70 percent of all women after delivery.

Postpartum Blues

Symptoms of maternal blues are frequent crying episodes, mood swings, and feelings of sadness, low energy, anxiety, insomnia, restlessness, and irritability. Women who experience these feelings should feel comforted that these feelings are normal and will pass on their own in a couple of weeks. Maternal blues are most likely caused by the enormous hormonal shifts in your body following delivery. An enormous lifestyle shift may also trigger these feelings due to an increase in stress and responsibility, worry about your newborn, physical discomfort associated with your postpartum physique, and possible exhaustion following labor and delivery.

Postpartum Depression (PPD)

Postpartum depression is a more serious and persistent condition that affects 10 to 15 percent of the postpartum population. Depression can begin at any time after delivery—from the first few hours afterward to a few weeks after. The symptoms include sadness, mood changes, lack of energy, loss of interest, change in appetite, fatigue, guilt, self-loathing, suicidal thoughts, and poor concentration and memory. When these feelings last for more than a couple of weeks, the consequences can be truly negative, leading to problems with bonding and relationship trouble. However, women don't go from the maternal blues to depression. In fact, you can feel well after delivery and then suddenly develop postpartum depression.

The causes of postpartum depression are possibly similar to those cited as causes for the milder maternal blues. But women at risk for this more serious depression are those with a family history of depression and women who have a poor support system at home (spouseless, bad relationship with partner, teenage mothers, and so on).

If you do begin to notice these feelings, treatment is available through counseling or therapy. Some women may require antidepressant medication combined with talk therapy. Above all, make sure that your TSH level has been checked by your doctor to be sure that you get the correct diagnosis and treatment.

Thyroid Disease in Newborns and Infants

An infant's brain *must* have a normal supply of thyroid hormone for it to grow and develop. This section discusses the effects of thyroid disease on the still-developing brain and body of newborns and infants. Normal thyroid levels are so important that newborn screening programs for thyroid disease are common practice in all industrialized countries, although sadly they are still not routine in many other parts of the world.

Hypothyroidism

In adults, the result of hypothyroidism can range from a minor annoyance that is easily remedied to a major medical problem with important, yet temporary, consequences. On the other hand, hypothyroid newborns and infants risk permanent mental retardation if thyroid hormone therapy is not started right away. Since iodine deficiency is a common cause of hypothyroidism in developing countries, the World Health Organization and a number of social service organizations have made iodine supplementation an international priority.

Newborn screening programs to detect hypothyroidism became practical in the 1970s and have become standard practice throughout the United States, Canada, and most industrialized countries. They use drops of blood, obtained by pricking the newborn's heel, spotted on filter paper. Special tests have been developed to measure T4 levels and TSH levels on the same dried blood spot. High TSH levels result in contacting the mother to begin thyroid hormone treatment for the baby. These screening techniques have nearly eliminated the severe mental retardation resulting from untreated congenital hypothyroidism in countries fortunate enough to have such programs.

It's important to start treatment with levothyroxine as soon as newborn hypothyroidism is discovered. Infants are started on a dosage between 37 and 50 mcg daily, adjusting the dosage according to the baby's response, the free T4 level, and the TSH level. It seems that the TSH level may stay slightly high despite appropriate levothyroxine treatment; however, this may be a sign that the baby is missing doses of T4.

Permanent Hypothyroidism

The majority of hypothyroidism cases detected by newborn screening are permanent, most resulting from abnormal formation of the thyroid gland (called thyroid dysgenesis). Two-thirds of newborns with thyroid dysgenesis have an ectopic thyroid, which means a thyroid gland in a different body location from the usual place.

During development of the embryo, the thyroid gland descends from the base of the tongue downward to the base of the neck, so the most common location for an ectopic thyroid is either at the tongue base or anywhere in the midline of the neck above the breastbone. Less commonly, thyroid glands may be found in the middle of the chest, sometimes even inside the heart or lower in the body. Ectopic thyroid glands are usually defective and unable to make much thyroid hormone, accounting for the infant's hypothyroidism; sometimes, however, they work well enough, making the discovery of a thyroid gland, appearing as a strawberry-like lump at the base of the tongue, a strange surprise during a dental examination.

A quarter of the time the baby is athyreotic, which means he or she hasn't any thyroid gland at all. This is likely due to a mutation in the embryo, where the genetic sequence involved with turning on other genes responsible for forming the thyroid gland is flawed. Less common are thyroids that are much smaller than normal (hypoplastic) and unable to make sufficient thyroid hormone.

Thyroid dyshormonogenesis is a term encompassing a variety of conditions in which the thyroid gland is unable to manufacture thyroid hormone. These conditions include: the inability to make iodine join onto proteins or amino acids, the inability to join together the components that make T3 and T4, the inability of the thyroid to respond to TSH, or the failure to take up iodine. Another condition resulting in thyroid dyshormonogenesis is called Pendred syndrome, a disorder characterized by deafness (caused by nerve dysfunction), goiter, and hypothyroidism from a mutation in the pendrin protein, which is responsible for some of the movement of iodine out of thyroid cells.

It's rare for newborns to have pituitary or hypothalamic problems as a cause of hypothyroidism. They usually occur together with malformations of facial and brain structures. In these conditions, blood tests show low total T4 levels with normal or low TSH levels. The same blood test results are seen when thyroxine-binding globulin (TBG) is deficient and the thyroid is actually normal, a condition seen much more frequently than pituitary or hypothalamic disease. This is because the screening tests only measure the total T4, which is low when TBG is absent, rather than the free T4, which is normal in TBG deficiency.

Transient Hypothyroidism

A variety of iodine-containing cleansing agents or contrast dyes used in x-ray imaging tests can be given to the mother during pregnancy or to the baby after birth. Excess iodine can inhibit the production of thyroid hormone by the baby's thyroid. This is more likely to happen in small or premature babies. Likewise, medications given to the mother for Graves' disease, such as methimazole or PTU, can block the baby's thyroid from making thyroid hormone. Since the effects of excess iodine and antithyroid drugs disappear when they're no longer around, they cause only transient hypothyroidism.

Antibodies from the mother that block the effects of TSH on its receptor can cause very rare cases of hypothyroidism in the baby. These antibodies are similar to the antibodies that cause Graves' disease by stimulating the TSH receptor, except that they have the opposite effect on the receptor. Since they've been present through much of the pregnancy, they may cause permanent deficiencies in brain development even though they gradually dissipate after birth.

Hyperthyroidism

Almost all of the time, hyperthyroidism in newborns is a temporary problem. The thyroid-stimulating antibodies that cause it are transferred through the placenta from the mother with Graves' disease. This is suspected when the newborn has an unexplained rapid heartbeat, a goiter, prominent eyes, irritability, poor weight gain, and a mother with active Graves' disease or a past history of Graves' disease. As in adults, PTU or methimazole, as well as the beta-blocker propranolol, are used to treat the baby since the antibodies may take a couple of months to go away.

Pediatric Thyroid Disease

Pediatric thyroid disease is also common but is not covered in this book. The range of thyroid problems we see in the adult population can be seen in children, particularly thyroid cancer, which appears to be on the rise in children. Mostly, the treatments are the same, but there are some nuances.

9

Hot Stuff

A Beginner's Guide to Radioactive Iodine

THIS CHAPTER FOCUSES on giving you a thorough explanation of the role of radioactive iodine (RAI) in treating thyroid disease and in scanning for diagnostic purposes. The mere thought of putting RAI into your body can be disturbing. Many of us have come to fear radioactive substances, sometimes correctly, as they have so many terrible historical associations: Hiroshima, Nagasaki, the Marshall Islands, Three Mile Island, and Chernobyl, just to name a few.

One reason thyroid patients worry about RAI is because of the misinformation they hear from other people—or even doctors. The most frightening aspect of RAI is that it's a very complicated substance to both explain and understand. You don't have to be a nuclear physicist to understand radioactive iodine, but it helps. When I was lecturing once at the National Graves' Disease Foundation, I started my talk with: "Who among us can claim to be a nuclear physicist?" One gentlemen did raise his hand and agreed that the patient literature on listserves and blogs has so distorted and exaggerated the perceived risks of RAI—especially for Graves' patients—that he felt that making informed decisions about it (for those of us who are not physicists) was next to impossible. This chapter is intended to clear up this misinformation and debunk common myths.

What Is Radioactive Iodine?

Radioactive iodine was discovered accidentally in the 1940s as a by-product of research carried out at the atomic laboratory in Oak Ridge, Tennessee. The adjective *radioactive* is used to describe elements containing unstable atoms—atoms that are emitting energy and hence releasing radiation. A radioactive form of any element is called a radioactive isotope, meaning an "unstable variety of this element." Imagine, for example, that you're trying to carry three hundred loose Ping-Pong balls in your arms from one end of a room to the other without dropping any. It's impossible. Inevitably, as you try to balance and juggle the balls, some will fall from your grip. Essentially, this is what happens when an element like iodine is radioactive. The iodine atoms can't securely grip the particles in their center. As a result, some of these subatomic particles are released, and the element is therefore unstable. But unlike the Ping-Pong balls, when these particles (energy) hit the "ground" (living tissue cells), they can damage and kill the cells.

If you're being treated for cancer, radiation and radioactive particles can be used in a positive way. In this case, the goal of the treatment is to deliberately damage your cancer cells to prevent them from reproducing and spreading throughout your body. To treat thyroid cancer, radioactive iodine is used because it is the thyroid's nature to actively take up this particular element, as has been explained throughout this book.

Historically, thyroid disease was the first type of illness in which radioactive substances proved essential for both diagnosis and treatment, providing the starting basis for the entire field of nuclear medicine. Radioactive iodine isotopes have played major roles in understanding the normal physiology of the thyroid and the nature of thyroid diseases, particularly in Graves' disease (Chapter 3), toxic multinodular goiters (see Chapter 5), and thyroid cancer (Chapter 6). The isotope typically used for scanning and treatment is known as either I-123 or I-131 (I is for iodine, and the number represents the number of neutrons in the isotopes).

RAI is used in small doses, ranging from 5 to 200 microcuries, to create scan images of the thyroid gland or measure the quantity of radioactive iodine taken up by the gland. Slightly larger doses of I-131, ranging from 1 to 5 millicuries (which equal 1,000 to 5,000 microcuries), are used to perform scans of the entire body after a cancer-containing thyroid gland is removed to look for thyroid cancer deposits. The doses of I-131 used to treat Graves' disease range from 4 to 30 millicuries. Thyroid cancer treatments use the highest doses of I-131, ranging from 30 to 200 millicuries for most situations and much higher doses (200 to 800 millicuries) for special situations with widespread tumors.

Nuclear Testing with Radioactive Iodine

Most people are first introduced to RAI through diagnostic testing. RAI is used to evaluate a range of thyroid conditions, particularly nodules (see Chapter 5) and thyroid cancer (see Chapter 6). You may not need an RAI scan, especially if you're hypothyroid. In fact, most of the thyroid scans that physicians order are unnecessary. This section discusses who is most likely to have an RAI scan and also covers when you should not have a scan.

RAI Uptake Tests

The RAI uptake test is most useful for evaluating thyrotoxicosis. If the uptake is high, then hyperthyroidism, usually from a toxic thyroid nodule or Graves' disease, will be seen as the cause of the excess thyroid hormone. If the uptake is low, then the cause of thyrotoxicosis is from excess ingestion of thyroid hormone or release of stored thyroid hormone from an inflamed thyroid gland (thyroiditis). If you have Graves' disease, your physician may use the RAI uptake result to calculate the amount of radioactive iodine needed to treat the hyperthyroidism.

Each thyroid cell takes up iodine to make thyroid hormone. The average thyroid gland weighs around 20 g, with each gram taking up around 1 percent of the iodine available from the diet. Usually, if the thyroid gland is stimulated and has become hyperthyroid, it takes up more iodine. Likewise, thyroid glands that are not working well and do not make thyroid hormone usually take up less iodine. To measure this, a person is given a small dose of radioactive iodine (I-123 or I-131) to swallow. One day later, a radiation detector is placed near the thyroid gland. The portion of the total dose of RAI that was swallowed that is measured in the thyroid gland is called the twenty-four-hour radioactive iodine uptake. Although a normal uptake is between 15 and 25 percent, this result can be greatly affected by the person's diet. People who eat foods that are high in iodine, such as iodized salt, dairy products, kelp, or seafood, will have a lower uptake. This is because, although their thyroid's ability to suck up iodine has not been altered, the nonradioactive dietary iodine dilutes out the portion of the RAI that goes into the thyroid gland, resulting in a lower uptake.

Radioactive Scans and Imaging

Radioactive isotopes concentrate within the thyroid gland or, in the case of thyroid cancer, in tumor cells spread anywhere in the body. In a radioactive scan, a radioactive isotope is administered by mouth and you're then placed in front of a machine that is able to detect the gamma rays (x-rays) that come from the radioactive isotope in the thyroid gland or in tumor cells. This machine puts together a picture or scan based on the x-ray "glows" coming from the person's body. There are a variety of types of scans as well as types of radioactive isotopes used to make these images.

Thyroid scans are used to see how much of the thyroid gland is taking up iodine, representing parts of the gland that are functioning normally, overfunctioning by taking up higher amounts of iodine ("hot" areas on the scan), or underfunctioning and not taking up iodine well ("cold" areas on the scan). To begin the test you will be given a small dose of a radioactive tracer, and the best tracer is the I-123 isotope of iodine. This is because using radioactive iodine for the scan best represents the natural processes of the thyroid gland, and I-123 exposes a person to less radiation than I-131, although I-123 is more expensive than I-131. Alternatively, many scans are done using an isotope of technetium, ^{99m}Tc. Technetium is most readily available to nuclear medicine departments and can provide a useful scan image; however, it does not always give the same picture as an iodine isotope scan.

When You Don't Need a Scan

If you are thyrotoxic (with a low TSH level and normal or high free T4), a thyroid scan can show whether the entire thyroid gland is overactive (hot) or there is a distinct nodule that is overactive. Many times, thyroid scans are used to evaluate thyroid glands with nodules, distinct lumps, or masses. This is only useful if the TSH level is low (less than 0.2), so that you can see if the nodule is hot or cold. A hot nodule (if the TSH is low) is known as a toxic thyroid nodule and is treated with radioactive iodine or surgery.

If the TSH level is not low, a scan should *not* be used to evaluate a thyroid nodule. This is because, no matter what the scan shows, it will not answer the critical question of whether the nodule is thyroid cancer. The only way that this question can be reliably answered, short of having surgery, is by a fine needle aspiration (FNA) biopsy (see Chapter 5). Sometimes thyroid scans are used inappropriately to check out the size of the thyroid gland or to look for nodules. This is best done by the physical examination or with an ultrasound of the thyroid gland.

RAI Whole Body Scans: For Thyroid Cancer Only

Radioactive iodine scans of the entire body are only used to evaluate you for thyroid cancer after you have had your thyroid gland removed by surgery. If you're reading this because you have thyroid cancer, make sure to read Chapter 6, which explains the basis for follow-up and scans.

To have an accurate whole body scan (WBS), you need to be prepared for it through a fairly elaborate process. First, you need to have a high TSH level (greater than 30) to stimulate thyroid and thyroid cancer cells. Next, you need to make sure that you eliminate as much iodine from your diet as possible so that the RAI scan is not ruined, because dietary iodine can interfere with the body's ability to suck up RAI. The amount of iodine in the average American diet exceeds the amount of iodine in the radioactive "tracer" dose by several hundred-fold and can dilute the uptake of the radioactive iodine, making the scan much less effective for detecting any cancer cells. You'll need to follow a low-iodine diet for at least two weeks, which is discussed in Chapter 11. A low-iodine diet improves the sensitivity of a WBS about tenfold. Third, you must avoid having a CT scan that uses contrast iodine dye. Fourth and finally, you must *not* be pregnant. Even if you don't think you can possibly be pregnant, you must have a pregnancy test before having any kind of RAI scan, including a WBS.

There are two methods of preparation for a WBS: the hypothyroid withdrawal method and the Thyrogen method. Regardless of the prep method used before a WBS, you'll need to be on the low-iodine diet.

Hypothyroid Withdrawal Preparation: The Classic Method

The classic, gold standard method of raising your TSH level is to just stop taking your thyroid hormone (levothyroxine). Until around 2001, this is what all thyroid cancer patients did before an alternative method became available. Withdrawing from your thyroid hormone takes about six weeks. To avoid hypothyroid symptoms for the first four weeks, you're given pure T3, which is sold as Cytomel, twice daily. This is one of the few situations in which you *must* take T3. Then you stop T3 and slowly become severely hypothyroid. You'll feel terrible because you'll have most of the symptoms discussed in Chapter 2. You *must* not drive while you are severely hypothyroid (meaning that your TSH is over 30).

One clear advantage to being made hypothyroid is that it enhances the sensitivity of the scan, since hypothyroid kidneys do not get rid of the radioactive iodine from the blood as rapidly as kidneys with normal thyroid hormone levels, which permits the RAI greater availability to be taken up by tumor cells. Because of this, no other current method of WBS preparation provides better sensitivity than the hypothyroid withdrawal method. Another advantage is that if any cancer is found, you can have treatment right away, as you'll need to be hypothyroid for treatment. This method is usually reserved for people who are having their first scans after thyroid surgery. If your scans are clean (meaning that they show no evidence of cancer), you can have an injection of artificially produced TSH, called *Thyrogen*, which means you do not have to be hypothyroid for your next scan. There is another version of the withdrawal method in which you are only moderately hypothyroid, but it's not recommended.

Thyrogen: Artificial TSH Injections Without Hypothyroidism

Thyrogen is an artificial thyroid-stimulating hormone, known by its generic name as recombinant human TSH (rTSH). You'll still need to be on a low-iodine diet for this prep method. Usually, Thyrogen is injected into the muscles of your arm or buttocks on the first and second days of a five-day period. On the third day, you swallow your I-131 tracer dose; on the fourth day, you have a blood test to measure the thyroglobulin level; and on the fifth day, you have your scan.

The advantage of this prep method is that you can be spared all the symptoms of hypothyroidism and can continue to drive and work. But there are also disadvantages. Thyrogen is very expensive and may not be covered by some insurance plans. Thyrogen does not have the same kidney effect as being hypothyroid; you'll lose RAI faster through your urine, meaning that it reduces the opportunity for tumor cells to suck up RAI and thus the scans may be less sensitive than those obtained using the classic method. Another disadvantage of Thyrogen is that many nuclear medicine departments use the same ten-minute scans for people getting Thyrogen scans as those getting hypothyroid withdrawal scans. *This may create false negatives, or clean scans, as Thyrogen scans require a longer scanning time.*

Most people will likely be offered Thyrogen unless they have not had clean scans (even then, many physicians will use Thyrogen again) or they have very aggressive tumors. Thyrogen was also recently approved for use by the FDA for ablation treatment with RAI for thyroid cancer.

Radioactive Iodine Treatment

Radioactive iodine, specifically I-131, has been used for treating thyroid disorders for more than half a century. It's used to treat cases of hyperthyroidism (see Chapter 3). It's also the mainstay of thyroid cancer treatment after the thyroid gland and the main thyroid cancer is removed by a surgeon. I-131 is dissolved in water. Sometimes this is added to gelatin capsules and swallowed, but it's preferable to take it in liquid form, sipping it through a straw. The actual amount of iodine that is swallowed is rarely more than a couple of milligrams, although it is usually quite radioactive.

You must not be treated with RAI if you're pregnant or breast-feeding. If you're pregnant, RAI will destroy the fetus's thyroid gland and expose it to unwanted radiation. If you're breastfeeding, you'll need to delay treatment for at least two months after you have completely weaned your baby. It will take that long for the breasts to completely stop making milk. Also, iodine concentrates in the breasts if they're filled with milk, which exposes your breasts to too much radiation.

RAI Ablation Treatment for Graves' Disease

RAI is an excellent treatment for Graves' disease. In North America, RAI is most frequently used to treat this condition, while in Europe and Japan, antithyroid drugs are used more often than RAI. For this reason, Graves' patients have wondered whether safety is the reason. It isn't. There are regional differences based on societal fears of RAI. In Europe and Japan, historical issues concerning nuclear bombs and testing weigh very heavily on patients' attitudes. These unfounded fears prolong suffering for many Graves' patients. RAI is used in Graves' disease to ablate, or destroy, the thyroid gland; stop your suffering; and make you permanently hypothyroid. This enables your doctor to put you on thyroid hormone to restore you to normal thyroid levels, making you feel normal again.

The iodine is given to you in liquid or gel cap form. There are different methods used to decide on the dosage of RAI, but 15 millicuries is the average dose for Graves' disease. Some physicians give arbitrary doses of I-131, knowing that most people will have some good results as long as the dose is reasonable (often around 10 millicuries). It is nearly impossible to reliably give a precise dose of RAI to allow a Graves' patient to be left with normal thyroid gland function. If someone promises you this, it's a sign either that he or she is inexperienced or that you may not have heard right. What physicians frequently say is that you'll feel normal "for a while" but will eventually become hypothyroid. Most thyroid experts feel it's best to give a dose that makes you hypothyroid as soon as possible so that you can start on thyroid hormone and get on with your life. (See Chapter 3 for more on treatment approaches for Graves' disease.)

It takes from one to four months before the RAI has had sufficient time to do all that it will do. Thyroid hormone levels should be monitored every three to five weeks until it is clear that you need thyroid hormone treatment (see Chapter 10). About one-third of the time, a second treatment with I-131 is needed. It's very rare to need a third treatment.

Hypothyroidism Following RAI for Graves' Disease

The intention of RAI ablation treatment is to destroy the thyroid gland, make you hypothyroid, and restabilize you on thyroid hormone so you feel "balanced" and well again. This is preferable to the roller coaster of thyrotoxicosis from Graves' disease (see Chapter 3), which wreaks havoc on your body—and life. Hypothyroidism should be seen not as a side effect but as a goal of treatment. If hypothyroidism is a surprise to you, or if you think it is a mistake, you do *not* have the right information and probably did not have informed consent.

Masha's Story: My Eight-Year Graves' Treatment

When I was diagnosed with Graves' disease, I joined a listserve and was warned about U.S. doctors pushing RAI on me, that it could cause cancer and ruin my thyroid gland forever. This all scared me, and I wanted to just take the antithyroid medications. It didn't work well, and I would go into periods where I was too high and then had to take beta-blockers. This went on for about eight years, and I was told that I just had a very severe case of Graves' disease. Finally, I agreed to the RAI ablation therapy. In six months, I was hypothyroid, which we planned, and then I started on thyroid hormone and felt, finally, *well*. I am angry with myself for having waited, because it wasted precious years for me.

Radioactive Iodine for Autonomous Toxic Nodules

Autonomous toxic nodules (ATN), discussed in Chapter 5, either alone or as part of a toxic multinodular goiter, are also sometimes treated with RAI. The doses of RAI used for these nodules are slightly higher than those used for Graves' disease, but they are far lower than the doses used for thyroid cancer. Toxic nodules larger than 5.0 cm are usually best treated with surgery.

RAI Treatment for Thyroid Cancer

RAI treatment is the only effective treatment for papillary and follicular thyroid cancers once they have spread beyond the thyroid gland. It is the only known effective systemic (bodywide) thyroid cancer treatment; it can kill thyroid cancer cells in the entire body, wherever they may be hiding. This is necessary because many thyroid cancers can spread to multiple sites in the neck or distantly to the lungs or bones long before they are discovered in your thyroid gland. In addition, the smallest tumor deposit that can be seen by a human eye contains more than a million cancer cells. This means that a surgeon is incapable of reliably providing a cure by surgery, making the surgery only the first step of your treatment. I-131 therapy becomes the second step of your treatment because it is an effective systemic treatment for thyroid cancers that suck up iodine.

RAI is given in the same way that it is administered for Graves' disease, either as a liquid that's sipped through a straw or in capsules that are swallowed. The major difference is in the dose, which is much higher than the dose for Graves' disease. Because there are concerns about exposing other people who come in contact with you after your treatment to unnecessary radiation, there are posttreatment precautions you'll need to follow to protect those around you. If you're traveling through airports, you must have a doctor's letter that explains you have had RAI.

Preparing for RAI Treatment of Thyroid Cancer

A major difference between RAI treatment for Graves' disease or ATNs and RAI treatment for thyroid cancer is that you'll need to

Angela's Story: My Post-9/11 Therapy

I had my RAI treatment at Sloan/Kettering [in New York] and lived in Chicago. On my way home, I was going through JFK airport security and set off the radiation detector. I was stopped and searched, and it was pretty scary. I explained that I had had this treatment and showed them a letter that my doctor wrote, and they let me go, but it was the first time they had heard of this. It was really important that I had that doctor's letter!

be prepped before treatment for thyroid cancer via a method similar to the ones used for whole body scans (see page 141). You'll need to have high TSH levels of 30 or more, and you'll need to follow the low-iodine diet. Either the hypothyroid withdrawal method or the Thyrogen method discussed earlier can be used to prepare for treatment.

Radioactive iodine treatment is most effective if it is used on the smallest remains of thyroid cancer deposits after surgery has removed all evident tumors. If large (more than 0.5 in.) lumps of thyroid cancer are present, radioactive iodine, no matter how high the dose, is often unable to destroy them. The best results are seen when the surgeon has performed a thorough removal of all obvious thyroid cancer as well as all portions of the thyroid gland. This should be done before performing I-131 scans or treatments.

Standard Dosing

Low doses of RAI, such as those used for Graves' disease, are ineffective for treating thyroid cancer. Some thyroid cancer patients are given several low doses of 29.9 millicuries, for example, which usually doesn't work. Standard RAI doses for thyroid cancer are at least 100 millicuries when the thyroid cancer does not extend beyond the limits of the thyroid gland, there is no evidence of any metastases (spread of the cancer to body regions beyond the thyroid gland), and the type of thyroid cancer is not particularly aggressive. If the original thyroid surgery shows that cancer cells have spread to lymph nodes in the neck or if the RAI whole body scan (performed immediately before the RAI therapy) shows spots of I-131 in the neck, outside of the place where the thyroid gland used to be (the thyroid bed), the typical RAI dose is 150 millicuries. If the scans reveal that the thyroid cancer has spread outside of the neck, such as to the lungs, liver, or bones, standard doses are usually inadequate to deal with these tumors. While some physicians give 200-millicurie doses for such situations, they are best dealt with by using the maximum doses of I-131 that can be safely given without causing intolerable side effects, using a method called *dosimetry*, a method of safely figuring out the limits for maximum dose RAI therapy. This involves a complex process that is only available at a handful of medical centers in the world.

What Are the Side Effects?

The word *radioactive* makes people think of radiation sickness when they think about RAI. In fact, RAI causes very few side effects for most people. The side effects that are reported are a nuisance but are not serious health hazards. They include:

• **Decreased saliva.** RAI can affect the salivary glands, causing diminished or loss of saliva. Taking frequent small sips of water while eating can help deal with this.
• **Increased risk of tooth decay.** If you have loss of saliva, then you're at risk for tooth decay. This is because saliva is critical for washing food particles off teeth after eating. Carry a small toothbrush kit in your pocket or purse, and try to brush after every meal.
• **Salivary stones.** This refers to the swelling of one or more salivary glands (located under the ears and under the lower jaw) due to partial blockage of the salivary ducts by dried saliva. While it may seem like a tumor or an enlarged lymph node, it isn't. This problem usually responds to swishing warm liquid (water, tea, coffee, broth) in the mouth while gently massaging the swollen salivary gland. Usually, there is a sudden sour taste as the stale saliva is released, then the swelling goes away. If this does not work or if it is rapidly and frequently recurrent, then it is important to go to your doctor. Usu-

Carlos's Story: Concerns About RAI

When I was supposed to have radioactive iodine treatment for my thyroid cancer, I was going out of town to a specialist, but I also kept seeing my family doctor. My family doctor was very concerned for me and warned me that all my children and my wife could get cancer if they were around me after my treatment. He told me that I needed to take my family to a hotel for three weeks after my treatment and not see them. This was a real blow to my family, as they were already really worried. When I told my wife, she started to cry. In the end, I was going to check in to a hotel myself for three weeks. When I told my specialist about this, he got really furious with my family doctor and called him right away to explain that he was panicking over nothing and that to tell me this is just wrong advice and bad medicine. Anyway, I'm glad in the end that my specialist intervened. My family doctor later apologized and said that he should have read up on this more before telling me this. All I really needed to do, in the end, was to act like I had strep throat and keep a safe distance from people. I didn't need to live somewhere else and worry like that.

ally this problem happens several times within a few weeks and then doesn't happen for a long time.

• **Watering of the eyes.** Rarely, thyroid cancer patients develop a constant watering of their eyes. This seems to be related to a blockage of the tear duct that drains tears into the nose. A physician can often repair this by opening up this duct.

Getting Clearance

Large doses of radioactive iodine require you to be isolated in a private hospital room. Once your levels of radiation are safe enough for others to be exposed to you, you're allowed to go home, so long as you practice the following posttreatment precautions for the next fourteen days:

- Do not exchange bodily fluids with anyone (no sex, wet kissing, sharing utensils, and so on).
- Urinate while sitting (instead of standing, if you're a male).
- While you may use normal eating utensils and dishes, you must rinse them before anyone else handles them.
- Dispose of your toothbrush after fourteen days.
- Try to place a little bit of distance between yourself and others. One useful technique is to imagine that you have strep throat; the distance that others should keep from you would be similar.
- Do not sleep in the same bed as others for these fourteen days.
- Do not operate a motor vehicle for at least ten days, because the thyroid hormone that was restarted on discharge takes a while to start working.

Be Informed:
Misconceptions About Radioactive Iodine

A lot of fear-mongering has gone on with respect to posttreatment, or radiation safety, precautions, and there are many misconceptions about RAI in general. Here's a tour of common statements you may read on the Internet:

- **RAI therapy for Graves' disease is bad because it causes permanent hypothyroidism.** The end goal of RAI therapy for Graves' disease is to become hypothyroid. No one should be advised that the thyroid gland will be normal after RAI therapy. In short, people with Graves' disease who are surprised to learn that they are hypothyroid did not have full information about RAI treatment for Graves' disease from their doctors prior to consenting to this therapy. If you're hypothyroid, it's good news: the RAI therapy worked, and you will no longer suffer from the harmful effects of hyperthyroidism and thyrotoxicosis.

- **RAI therapy for Graves' disease causes thyroid cancer.** Many Graves' disease patients are concerned that RAI therapy will cause thyroid cancer or thyroid nodules later in life. Although this is a reasonable concern, it isn't the case, a fact based on over 50 years of study and observation.

- **Radioactive iodine causes birth defects.** The incidence of birth defects following RAI treatment has been thoroughly studied over the more than half-century that RAI has been used. To date, there's no evidence that RAI treatments cause any birth defects in babies of women who've completed RAI therapy before their pregnancy. On the other hand, you must be absolutely certain that you're not pregnant before treatment, as the RAI would go directly to the fetal thyroid gland and cause severe damage to the fetus. For more information on pregnancy and thyroid disease, see Chapter 8.

- **Radioactive iodine causes thyroid eye disease.** This is not the case for most Graves' patients in light of the use of steroid treatments. See Chapter 7 for more information.

- **Radioactive iodine is used more in the United States because it's cheaper, not safer.** The higher use of RAI in the United States as compared to Europe and Japan has to do with sociocultural issues, not safety, as discussed in the section "RAI Ablation Treatment for Graves' Disease" in this chapter.

- **RAI causes other cancers.** Many people treated for Graves' disease are concerned about the fact that RAI could increase their risks of getting other cancers. The two most common cancers rumored to be linked to RAI are leukemia and breast cancer.

With respect to leukemia, even with a single dosage of higher than 800 millicuries of radioactive iodine, far fewer than 1 out of 1,000 people on that extraordinarily high dosage might go on to develop leukemia. This incidence, however, could not be absolutely linked to RAI and might be expected as a risk in the population in anyone, unrelated to RAI.

With respect to breast cancer, a study published in 2000 showed an association between women under forty who been diagnosed with thyroid cancer and an increased incidence of breast cancer. The study, conducted by Amy Chen, M.D., M.P.H., of the University of Texas M.D. Anderson Cancer Center in Houston, found that women under forty who had thyroid cancer are more likely to develop breast cancer later in life compared to women who have not had thyroid cancer. No study, to date, has identified how thyroid cancer predisposes a woman to have breast cancer. Although it is tempting to speculate that this could be related to RAI treatment, there is no evidence of this link. Nonetheless, it's important to realize that treatment of a known cancer is more important than worries of a greater risk for a second cancer that is still unlikely to occur.

- **Radioactive iodine causes your hair to fall out.** Hair loss during and after the hypothyroid preparation for radioactive iodine scanning or therapy is caused by the changes in thyroid hormone status. It is completely unrelated to the radioactive iodine or to any radiation effect. All such hair loss is completely replaced by natural growth when the thyroid hormone levels are restored.

10

Helping the Medicine
Go Down

Thyroid Hormone Replacement
and Other Medications

FOR THE MAJORITY of thyroid disorders discussed in this book, all paths lead to thyroid hormone replacement. If you're hypothyroid (see Chapter 2) for any reason, you'll need to take thyroid hormone to restore your thyroid hormone levels to normal. If you're hyperthyroid as a result of Graves' disease, and your thyroid gland is ablated with radioactive iodine or allowed to burn out (see Chapters 3 and 9), you'll eventually wind up hypothyroid and will need to take thyroid hormone to restore your thyroid hormone levels to normal. Finally, if you've had a total thyroidectomy to treat thyroid cancer or for any other reason, you'll be hypothyroid and will require thyroid hormone replacement as well. Thyroid cancer patients will actually require what's known as TSH suppression therapy. With the exception of transient hypothyroidism from thyroiditis (see Chapter 4), thyroid hormone therapy is medicine you'll need for life.

Unfortunately, there is a lot of misinformation about thyroid hormone replacement therapy. Some of it can lead thyroid patients into taking bizarre supplements they don't need. There is also confusion over which thyroid hormone to take: T4, which is levothyroxine, the hormone that your thyroid naturally makes and converts into triiodothyronine (T3), or pure T3, typically sold under the brand name Cytomel. This chapter will give you the correct information about all the formulations of thyroid hormone and address the misinformation you may have read.

A Brief History of Thyroid Hormone Replacement

In 1891 an extract of sheep thyroid successfully treated severe hypothyroidsm (known as myxedema) in a forty-six-year old woman, who then lived an additional twenty-eight years. And thus was born a wonderful therapy for thyroid disease: desiccated (dried) animal thyroid extract. During the 1890s medical textbooks provided recipes for preparing animal thyroid glands; one recipe, for example, was for fried, minced thyroid served with bread and currant jelly for breakfast.

In 1927 synthetic levothyroxine (T4) was invented, but it was so expensive to produce that it was not widely available until better ways to produce it were invented in the 1960s. By then both T4 and T3 (triiodothyronine) were readily available, both as separate tablet preparations and as combined tablets. At first the combined tablets were standard of care. But during the 1970s researchers figured out that the extra T3 was not necessary because the body simply converted the T4 into T3; this led to better results as fewer people suffered from thyrotoxicosis. As for the animal thyroid hormone, prions (infectious agents) and purity issues were a concern. Since the 1970s, T4 therapy has emerged as the state-of-the-art treatment. These days, giving someone dried animal thyroid hormone is considered an outdated form of therapy.

Synthetic Versus "Natural" Thyroid Hormone: A Reality Check

Many patients read that levothyroxine sodium, which is a chemically pure copy of T4, is bad because it is synthesized in a lab. But, in fact, all thyroid hormone preparations are prepared in a lab, including dessicated pig thyroid hormone, which is falsely touted as "more natural." Make no mistake: the word *natural* is a marketing term;

similarly, the word *synthetic* is the term used by salespeople selling "natural" products to steer you away from the competition. The situation has gotten so absurd that in the thyroid world, patient advocates claim that pig thyroid hormone is more natural because it's derived from an animal, while in the menopause world, patient advocates want the estrogen equivalent of levothyroxine sodium (what they call "bioidentical hormones") because they claim that estrogen made from horse urine is synthetic. Meanwhile, thyroid patients claim that the human copy of the T4 hormone (levothyroxine) is synthetic, while menopause patients claim that the human copy of the estrogen hormones (compounded hormones from plants) is natural. It's clear that something is wrong with patient advocacy literature, which is confusing to thyroid patients trying to make sense of hormone information they read—especially thyroid patients who are perimenopausal.

The fact is that dessicated pig thyroid hormone is less natural to your body than levothyroxine sodium, which copies nature and human thyroid activity.

Be Informed: Synthetic T4

You may have heard the following statement: "Synthetic T4 is not as good as natural thyroid hormone or T3/T4 mixtures." This statement is false on several levels. First, all thyroid hormone preparations are synthetic in that they are synthesized in a lab. In the case of T4, this hormone is created by a pharmaceutical manufacturer using chemical reactions. This is similar to the way in which aspirin is made from willow tree bark or penicillin is made from mold. Making a drug or hormone in this way permits a pure, properly measured, and reproducible drug that is free of natural contaminants such as viruses, bacteria, or prions.

Dried thyroid animal hormone is falsely touted as "natural" for marketing purposes, but it contains many impurities and does not "copy nature" the way T4 does. Meanwhile, T3's short half-life of a day makes it unstable, meaning that your hormone levels could be unstable or inconsistent.

More About Dried Animal Thyroid Hormone

As mentioned earlier, from the nineteenth century until the 1960s, dried animal thyroid hormone was the standard of care. It was a preparation of dried, cleaned, powdered thyroid glands from sheeps, cows, or pigs. Sheep and cow thyroid hormone is no longer around, but pig thyroid hormone is still made, sold under the brand name Armour. However, pig thyroid hormone is *no longer* the standard of care because it contains a variety of hormones and chemicals from thyroid glands that are nearly impossible to accurately standardize from batch to batch. These hormones include T4, T3, thyroglobulin, and by-products of T3 with fewer iodine atoms on each molecule (T1 and T2). This means that dried pig thyroid hormone does not give you a stable potency; some batches are more potent than others. As in other areas of medicine, thyroid hormone preparations have advanced over time; in the 1960s, researchers figured out a better way to make thyroid hormone that was always the same potency and

Dara's Story: "This Ain't Your Grandmother's Thyroid Hormone Therapy"

When I researched thyroid hormone online, I came to the conclusion that the dried pig thyroid hormone, Armour, was what knowledgeable doctors prescribed, and that the outdated therapy was [levothyroxine sodium]. Hundreds of people on thyroid listserves say this. So I went on it, but my TSH test results were never consistent. I eventually moved to a different state and saw a very good endocrinologist who explained that Armour was the therapy my grandmother would have been on, but that I didn't need "my grandmother's thyroid hormone" since we got a lot smarter and figured out a lot more about stable thyroid hormone dosing. She switched me to levothyroxine sodium, and my TSH tests started to be consistent finally.

always stable—yet also affordable. This was done to make patients feel better.

Thyroid patient advocates frequently claim that more modern formulations of thyroid hormone do not work in all people. They also claim that these formulations are part of a pharmaceutical conspiracy to financially exploit patients and that thyroid doctors who prescribe levothyroxine are part of this conspiracy. These types of statements are not only absurd but also a warning sign that the source of these statements is ignorant about how the field of medicine works. Unfortunately, there is a cultlike pressure to take Armour thyroid over levothyroxine as a political act.

Twenty-First-Century Thyroid Hormone Therapy

Thyroid patients living in the twenty-first century ought to be offered twenty-first-century thyroid hormone therapy, not nineteenth-century therapy, as in animal thyroid hormone, or mid-twentieth-century therapy, as in the mixture of T3/T4. This doesn't mean that historic versions of therapy will necessarily harm you, but it does mean that you're not getting the modern standard of care when you take either pig thyroid hormone or a mixture of T3/T4 (see "Combination Therapy" later in this chapter).

Be Informed: The Truth About "Natural" Thyroid Hormone

Some websites say dried pig thyroid hormone is better because it contains "all four thyroid hormones: T1, T2, T3, and T4." T1 and T2 are what T4 degrades into; they have no activity, thus offering absolutely no benefit to you and are considered impurities that interfere with activity. They are analogous to a bicycle without wheels.

The remainder of this chapter will discuss T4, since it's the standard of care that you should be offered.

T4: Brand Names Versus Generics

A generic drug is a pill made to contain the same chemical form of the medication as a branded pill. Ideally, it should be identical to the name-brand version. With some types of medicine, the generic form of the drug is close enough to the original that it can be used just as well, which usually means it is less expensive and sometimes preferred by health insurance plans. The essential differences between some name-brand medications and their respective generic forms have to do with the quality control of the manufacturer, as well as the way that the tablet is put together, meaning the filler substances and dyes it contains. This quality control determines whether you end up with the proper amount of T4 in your blood and whether you can count on the same accurate dose the next time you go to the pharmacy and purchase a new batch of medication.

Thyroid hormone has a narrow therapeutic index. This means that very small differences in the amount of active T4 taken will result in significant differences in how it works in your body. This can be measured in a TSH test. For many years, doctors have seen changes in TSH levels from generics to brands. For this reason, thyroid experts recommend that you choose a reputable brand of T4 and stay on that brand. While various brands of T4 may be pharmacologically equivalent, TSH tests show that brands are not biologically equivalent. People feel differently on different brands and may require different dosing, according to brands. For the average hypothyroid patient, this may not be all that significant a difference. If you are a thyroid cancer patient requiring TSH-suppression therapy, however, it does make a difference. In this group of patients, very small differences in T4 pills can easily shift them from being "just right" to having too much or too little.

No Substitutes

Depending on your health plan, pharmacists can give you the cheapest version of T4, even if it's a generic, if this is a cost savings to your insurance company; sometimes this practice results in a greater profit margin for the pharmacy. Less frequently, the cost savings are passed on to you through lower prices. Sometimes the copayments on your insurance-subsidized prescription end up costing you more than the retail price if you choose not to use your insurance. The best advice from thyroid experts is to simply request that your doctor write "no substitutes" on the prescription once you find the brand that works best for you.

Dosing T4: One Size Does Not Fit All

Levothyroxine pills now come in a wide range of strengths so that dosing can be highly individualized. All of these pills, within the same brand, are the same physical size and shape, but there is a considerable difference in the amount of T4 contained in each pill. They range from 25 mcg (0.025 mg) to 300 mcg (0.3 mg), including:

50 mcg (0.05 mg)	125 mcg (0.125 mg)
75 mcg (0.075 mg)	137 mcg (0.137 mg)
88 mcg (0.088 mg)	150 mcg (0.15 mg)
100 mcg (0.1 mg)	175 mcg (0.175 mg)
112 mcg (0.112 mg)	200 mcg (0.2 mg)

There's such a wide variety of pill strengths that you shouldn't need to cut pills in half or take different size pills on different days. Sometimes, however, thyroid patients do need to be on unusual dosages, in which they may combine pills to get the right dosages, such as:

162 mcg = 112 mcg + 50 mcg
187 mcg = 112 mcg + 75 mcg
224 mcg = 112 mcg + 112 mcg
250 mcg = 125 mcg + 125 mcg

Although the pharmacist is supposed to label the bottle with the strength (or dosage) of the pill, it's best to be familiar with your pills by their appearance. Each strength of pill should have a characteristic color and identification number on it. This is particularly important considering that tens of thousands of pharmacist errors are made every year.

The average dose of T4 for a hypothyroid person is 1.6 mcg of T4 per kilogram of body weight per day. There is, however, a wide variation. The best way to find out the proper dose for you is to take a reasonable dosage T4 tablet (near to the average amount) every day for at least six weeks, then have your physician check your TSH level. If the TSH level is between 0.5 and 2.0, then you are on the correct T4 dose. If the TSH level is higher, your dose needs to be increased and the TSH level rechecked in six more weeks. If the TSH level is lower, then a slight reduction in the T4 dose would be appropriate; this should also be verified with a TSH level test after at least six weeks.

Thyroid cancer patients, who need to keep their TSH levels at around 0.1, average 2.0 mcg T4 per kilogram body weight per day. Dose adjustments are made in the same way as described above.

Storage and Heat Sensitivity

Although this is not common knowledge to pharmacists or doctors, T4 is very sensitive to heat. A good rule of thumb is to use "chocolate bar" rules: if the temperature is warm enough to soften a milk chocolate bar, then it will cause the T4 pill to go bad fairly quickly. Although the pill will look OK, it will not work well, providing far less T4 to you than a fresh pill. Don't keep your T4 pills on a shelf above the stove, leave your pills on the seat of your car on a summer afternoon, or carry your pill bottle in your purse. If you live in a hot climate without air conditioning, keep your pills in the refrigerator.

This problem can also occur in the drugstore or, if you have your pills delivered, during transport. Thyroid experts have noted the trend of high TSH levels in the summer and lower TSH levels in the winter.

Even with optimal storage conditions, T4 pills lose 5 percent of their potency each year. If you're on good terms with your pharmacist, ask him or her to check the expiration date on the stock bottle in the pharmacy. You don't want pills at the end of their shelf life. It's best to

Lionel's Story: Trucking Hypothyroid

My doctor kept accusing me of being a bad patient and not taking my thyroid pills because he said that I was hypothyroid. I kept telling my doctor it wasn't true and that I do take them. I'm a trucker and would keep my pills in the glove compartment and take them every morning—on an empty stomach— just like I was supposed to. I started to feel really hypo and got into a fender bender, which scared me. I went to see my doctor and asked if maybe there was something wrong with the pills. Finally, he figured out that the pills were probably bad from the heat. He started me on T3 because I was pretty hypo and needed to drive for work. He then put me on T4 at the same time. After about six weeks, I went off the T3 and felt OK. Now I keep my pills in a cooler when I'm on the road, with ice packs.

get the full 100-pill package, freshly sealed at the factory, rather than a monthly dispersal from a large T4 container of uncertain age.

How to Take Your T4

Start right with these simple rules:

• Take your T4 first thing in the morning on an empty stomach. Food in your stomach causes a slight decrease in the amount of T4 that is absorbed into your body. Even the slight delay between waking up and breakfast time is often sufficient to provide enough time for best absorption. Certain foods are more likely to interfere with T4 absorption; notable among them are liquid soy preparations. Hot liquids can also interfere with absorption, particularly coffee.
• **Stay consistent.** Take your pills at the same time each day.
• If you forget to take your morning dose, take it as soon as you can.

- If you miss your dose for the entire day, take two doses the next day to make up for it.
- If you miss multiple days, even up to a week, it is far safer to take all the missed pills at once than to miss the doses. (This can happen if you are traveling and encounter unexpected delays without having brought extra pills.)

Staying Consistent and Compliant

Remembering to take a pill every day and/or taking it correctly is known in pharmacy-speak as compliance. Some people take their daily T4 medication like clockwork, but most people are a bit forgetful. A useful device is a day-of-the-week pill container. These can be filled once a week and used to remind you to take your pill. Forgetting to regularly take T4 seems to be the most common reason for people to become hypothyroid while taking the same T4 dosages that were previously sufficient to bring their TSH to a normal level.

Children and elderly patients, who do not have full capacity to make medical decisions, may need to be monitored closely, as in all other cases in which they require lifelong medication.

Problems in Taking T4: Other Drugs/ Supplements That Interfere

T4 pills are completely absorbed within five hours of the time they are swallowed, and most of this takes place within the first three hours. The following may interfere with absorption:

- Iron, either as a supplemental medicine to treat iron deficiency or as part of a vitamin pill, will prevent T4 pills from being fully absorbed. If you need iron, take the first daily dose at least four hours after the T4 is taken. If you take vitamin pills that contain iron, take them at bedtime so that the T4 can be taken in the morning without interference.
- Some people need to take large daily doses of calcium. People with thyroid cancer who have suffered damage to their parathyroid glands frequently need this. If several calcium pills are taken at the

Kenisha's Story: Stranded in NOLA

I live in Tennessee but was in New Orleans to be with my mother when Hurricane Katrina hit in August 2005. She does not have great mobility and refused to leave. We went to the stadium in New Orleans to ride it out, which was supposed to be a safe zone for those of us who were there. We wound up stuck there for days on end without food, water, medical care, or help. I am hypothyroid and did not have enough pills. By the time I got out of there, I had gone about two weeks with no thyroid pills. When I got back home, I took seven pills all at once the first day back, and then another seven the second day, and then called my doctor to tell her what I did. She said that I may start to feel a bit jittery but that the half-life was so long, I would probably be okay, and I was. I saw a lot of people suffer without medications like insulin and heart pills and so forth. I actually felt lucky that I had some time to be without my meds without severe consequences.

same time as T4, then there might be some interference in absorption of the T4. Usually, as long as the T4 is taken immediately upon waking in the morning, the first calcium dose can be taken an hour or so later without much problem.

- Sucralfate, a drug used to coat your stomach to treat stomach irritation or ulcers, can also keep T4 from being absorbed into your body from your stomach.
- Cholestyramine and colestipol, drugs used to treat high cholesterol levels, can interfere with absorption.
- High doses of antacids (aluminum and magnesium hydroxides) are known to interfere with absorption.
- Liquid soy preparations, often used as milk substitutes or for baby formulas, can bind to T4 if taken in moderately large amounts within four hours of taking your T4 dose.

The Effects of Lithium

Lithium is prescribed for bipolar disorder. Even if your thyroid is functioning normally, lithium can cause hypothyroidism; 8 to 19 percent of people on lithium become hypothyroid. This can be a problem because the hypothyroidism can either cause depression or make your existing depression worse. This may result in an increased dosage of lithium, worsening the undiagnosed hypothyroidism. The best way to avoid this potential nightmare is to make sure your doctor checks your thyroid function. Then, insist that your thyroid levels be checked every six months while you're on lithium. In between checkups, you might want to keep a log of your moods on a day-to-day basis. If you're feeling unusually depressed for long periods of time, get your thyroid levels checked, just in case. Once you're on thyroid hormone, there is no more concern regarding lithium. It can only affect the production of thyroid hormone within the thyroid gland; it has no effect on how thyroid hormone acts in the rest of the body.

Lithium has also been known to cause goiters and hyperthyroidism and to trigger Graves' disease.

The Effects of Amiodarone

Amiodarone is a drug used to treat a heart rhythm problem. This drug contains a lot of iodine and has been found to induce both hypothyroidism and hyperthyroidism; in North America, where there is sufficient iodine, hypothyroidism is more common. In the United States, amiodarone can cause severe thyroiditis resulting in thyrotoxicosis that can last for several weeks. Amiodarone causes hyperthyroidism if you have a toxic multinodular goiter and live in an iodine deficient region. Since the drug is stored in body fat, it can induce a thyroid problem up to twelve months after you have discontinued using it.

When You Must Take T3

As discussed earlier, T3 (called triiodothyronine, liothyronine sodium, or the brand name Cytomel) is the active form of thyroid hormone. As discussed in Chapter 1, only 20 percent of the thyroid hormone made by the thyroid gland is T3, while the rest is T4. Most of the T3 in each cell of the body comes from T4 that has been converted into T3 while inside that cell. The reason you're given T4 is to copy nature, allowing each cell in your body to make its own T3, exercising some control over this by controlling the enzymes inside the cells that change T4 to T3. In some situations, you need to take only T3 and not T4.

People with Thyroid Cancer Preparing for RAI Therapy or Scans

For people with thyroid cancer who are preparing for a withdrawal whole body scan or a thyroglobulin test (see Chapter 9), a short course of T3 treatment is used when there is a need to make them hypothyroid (to raise the TSH to a level greater than 30) while minimizing hypothyroid symptoms. After having finished their radioactive iodine scan or therapy or after measuring their thyroglobulin level, another short course of T3 treatment can be used to restore their thyroid hormone levels faster, relieving hypothyroid symptoms and enabling them to go back to work and to drive again.

All drugs and hormones have limited times during which they can last inside the body. This is called the half-life. T3 has a very short half-life of one day, while T4 has a very long one of one week. One week after stopping T4, the T4 level is 50 percent of the baseline level, and after two weeks, it's still active at about 25 percent. If you are severely hypothyroid and need a fast-acting thyroid hormone that goes to work right away, you need T3. For example, this would be the case for thyroid cancer patients who need to start hormone therapy after being severely hypothyroid, following their scans or therapies with RAI.

The difference in the half-lives of T3 and T4 provides some advantages and disadvantages. The advantage for T4 is that the levels of T4 remain rock-steady when it's taken daily. Especially for people with thyroid cancer, who need their TSH level suppressed to less than 0.1 all the time, their regular daily T4 dose can be adjusted to do what is needed without any significant ups or downs. The disadvantage of T4 is that when thyroid cancer patients need to prepare for a withdrawal method scan (see Chapter 9), it takes around six weeks of gradually worsening hypothyroidism before enough T4 is gone to make the TSH rise high enough for radioactive iodine scans or treatments. The advantage for T3 is that its short half-life lets you stop it for only a short time to get your T3 levels low enough to permit the TSH levels to rise. This lets people use T3 as a filler hormone when they stop T4, so it's a terrific option. Typically, T4 is stopped six weeks before a radioactive iodine whole body scan for checking on a person with thyroid cancer. For the first four weeks, T3 is taken twice daily (usually around 25 mcg each dose for the average-sized adult), preventing any symptoms of hypothyroidism during this time. During the two weeks off of T3 (the fifth and sixth weeks off T4), symptoms of hypothyroidism begin quickly and the pituitary gland is able to make high enough TSH levels. This stimulates any thyroid cancer cells still around to reveal themselves by sucking up radioactive iodine during the scan or by producing thyroglobulin that can be measured in the blood.

In much the same way, but in reverse, the weeklong half-life of T4 means that it takes six weeks of daily T4 pills before hypothyroid people with thyroid cancer can restore their T4 level to their usual baseline. Many thyroid cancer experts use T3, in gradually decreasing dosages, to help people feel better faster, in combination with T4 for the first three weeks. After the radioactive iodine scan or treatment is done, patients start their usual daily T4 dose. For the first week, they supplement this with a twice-daily T3 pill (usually a 25 mcg pill for the average adult); for the second week, they take half a T3 pill twice daily; and for the third week, they take half a T3 pill to get started each morning. By the end of the third week of resuming the thyroid hormone, the T4 level (although not yet at the final level) is high enough to prevent them from having more than minimal hypothyroid symptoms and they can stop the T3.

T3 for Severe Hypothyroidism

In rare situations, someone may be found to be severely hypothyroid, which can even lead to a myxedema coma. In these instances, pure

T3 needs to be given along with T4 to get the active hormone into the person quickly; in fact, T3 is sometimes given intravenously. The person will then need to begin taking long-acting T4, which will get the body to convert T4 into T3 naturally.

Combination Therapy: Why Do Doctors Prescribe It?

One reason doctors do not prescribe T3 as a usual thyroid hormone replacement therapy is precisely because the half-life is so short. This creates a "peak and valley" effect for hypothyroid people, who will spend half the day slightly thyrotoxic and the other half slightly hypothyroid. This is not good therapy.

Another disadvantage of pure T3 is that it bypasses the natural body processes that regulate and customize the amount of T3 produced in each cell from T4. Researchers have shown that T4 is more easily transported from the blood into the brain than T3 and that brain cells (neurons) are best suited to respond to T3 made from T4 entering their support (glial) cells or entering the neurons directly. Right now, the best medical and physiological knowledge shows pure T4 pills to be the appropriate way to treat hypothyroid people.

So, what about combination T3/T4? Since the thyroid gland normally releases 80 percent of its thyroid hormone as T4 and 20 percent as T3, it seems logical to make a tablet that combines T4 and T3 in a similar ratio. Some pills are manufactured that do just that. Unfortunately, this type of pill cannot do the same thing as a normal thyroid gland that releases a constant, steady stream of both hormones all day and night. Instead, the pill releases both the T4 and T3 completely over one to three hours. This is far from the natural state of affairs and causes unnatural ups and downs of thyroid hormone. Nonetheless, some physicians prescribe these pills for hypothyroid people, and some people say they feel better on a combination dose.

Several randomized control trials have been done to determine whether people really do feel better on the combination therapy or if this is due to the placebo effect. The results of eleven randomized controlled trials, including one thorough metanalysis (where researchers looked at all the trials to see if they were designed correctly and recalculated results), have found that people do no better on the combination therapy, and, in fact, some may be a little thyrotoxic on the combination therapy. Many physicians say they prescribe combination therapy to patients because the patients request it and, in most cases, it won't harm them. Eventually, most of these patients wind up going back to T4, especially after bouts of instability on T3/T4. If you're reading this and wondering if combination therapy is for you, the answer according to the scientific evidence to date is no.

11

What to Eat

Diet, Nutrition, and Thyroid Disease

THERE IS NO such thing as a "thyroid diet," but diet plays a critical role in thyroid health. This chapter discusses the role of dietary iodine in maintaining thyroid health and the role of low-iodine diets for thyroid cancer patients. This chapter also addresses hypothyroidism and weight gain, as well as the range of dietary habits that can combat constipation and poor energy. Finally, this chapter discusses the role obesity plays in thyroid disease.

Diet and Iodine

As discussed in Chapter 1, the thyroid gland extracts iodine from various foods to make thyroid hormone. Your thyroid gland will use about a milligram of iodine per week (150 mcg per day) to make thyroid hormone; that is a tiny amount, so a balanced diet provides more than enough iodine for the average thyroid gland. A healthy thyroid gland is designed to take what it needs from your daily diet, and it can store enough iodine to last for three months. Given that the thyroid gland needs such a small amount of iodine to do its work, it seems unlikely that iodine deficiency would be a problem. But it is; a healthy thyroid gland suffers without sufficient quantities of iodine. On the other hand, there are therapeutic reasons why being on a low-iodine diet is critical, as is the case for thyroid cancer patients preparing for radioactive iodine therapies or scans.

Iodine Deficiency and the Thyroid

Without enough iodine in the diet, the thyroid gland cannot produce thyroid hormone. When this happens, the pituitary gland makes more TSH, continuing to stimulate the thyroid gland and causing it to enlarge, a condition called a goiter. Most people need about 150 mcg of iodine each day to produce enough thyroid hormone and avoid developing a goiter. Unfortunately, much of the world's population lives in goiter belts—regions that have very low levels of iodine in the soil and water.

Without iodine supplements, people living in goiter belts consume insufficient iodine to maintain their health. If this deficiency is severe, newborn children can suffer from mental retardation, short stature, hypothyroidism, and goiters; these symptoms together are called cretinism. Even in the absence of all the signs of cretinism, low iodine levels are responsible for decreased brain development and mental retardation; this is because the lack of iodine reduces the level of thyroid hormone during early development.

In regions with low levels of iodine in the diet, the reduction in mental abilities of its people contributes to poor social and economic productivity and is partly responsible for poverty and underdevelopment. Most mountainous areas of the world, such as the Andes Mountains, the Himalayas, portions of mainland China, the Alps, central Mexico, and much of Greece, are iodine deficient. Large iodine-deficient areas of the world also include northern and central Africa, the interior of Brazil, and the Netherlands. In most of the industrialized portions of the world, aggressive efforts to provide iodine supplementation have significantly reduced this deficiency. Many decades ago, for example, the Great Lakes region of the United States was a goiter belt, but this is no longer so. For the rest of the world, however, this remains a major problem with significant health and social consequences.

In fact, over one billion people are at risk for iodine deficiency–related thyroid disease. Two hundred million people suffer from goiters, while twenty million people suffer from brain damage due to iodine deficiency during pregnancy and infancy. This is very disturbing, since these problems can be completely prevented by the simple addition of iodized salt or iodized oil (proposed in some regions) to the diet.

The first International Goiter Congress was held in 1929 in Bern, Switzerland, after Switzerland and the United States introduced iodized salt. Many countries soon followed suit, and iodine deficiency has disappeared in most parts of the world. However, not much happened to eliminate iodine deficiency in underdeveloped nations until 1985, when thyroid specialists established the International Council for Control of Iodine Deficiency Disorders (ICCIDD), a group of about four hundred members from seventy countries.

In North America, only about one in four thousand newborns is born with hypothyroidism; in iodine-deficient areas, 10 percent of all newborns are hypothyroid. Worse, up to 70 percent of the iodine-deficient populations are severely hypothyroid. As a result, iodine deficiency is now recognized as the most common cause of preventable mental defects. ICCIDD works with the World Health Organization and UNICEF to develop national programs in Africa, Asia, Latin America, and Europe with the goal of eliminating iodine deficiency in our lifetime. Most recently, the salt industry has joined in the fight too.

Can an Iodine-Rich Diet Prevent Thyroid Disease?

If you have a normally functioning thyroid gland but are concerned that you are at risk for a thyroid problem, can an iodine-rich diet prevent thyroid disease? It depends on where you live. We know that a lack of iodine can cause the thyroid gland to enlarge. However, too much iodine is believed to be responsible for triggering goiters and thyroid disorders as well. That's one reason why taking kelp (seaweed) is not recommended. If you live in North America, you're probably getting enough iodine in your diet from your food thanks to iodized salt. Taking kelp with the belief that it will prevent a thyroid problem is a bad idea. It may trigger a thyroid problem instead of preventing one.

In North America, except for advising you against taking kelp, physicians do not generally issue warnings to people at risk for a thyroid disorder about avoiding food containing iodine. That's because iodine is found in a host of different foods that offer important nutrients. Since iodine is present in so many foods, it's unlikely that someone will suffer from iodine deficiency in North America.

The Problem with Excess Iodine

In countries where iodine has been made plentiful in the food supply, such as in the United States, hypothyroidism from iodine deficiency has disappeared. However, hypothyroidism from autoimmune disease has skyrocketed.

It seems that excess iodine in the diet stimulates the immune system to create antibodies that attack the thyroid gland and cause it to stop making normal amounts of thyroid hormone, a condition called Hashimoto's thyroiditis (see Chapter 2). Also, among people who get thyroid cancer, iodine supplementation has changed the types of thyroid cancer, decreasing the proportion of follicular thyroid cancers and increasing the number of papillary thyroid cancers. The reasons why iodine supplementation does these things are unknown. In healthy people who take very high doses of iodine once in a while, such as using iodine-containing water-purification tablets on a camping trip, excess iodine temporarily shuts off the thyroid gland and reduces its production of thyroid hormone. However, healthy thyroids will usually regain the ability to make thyroid hormone despite continued exposure to high iodine levels.

Be Informed: The Myth About Herbal Supplements

In general, herbs that are marketed for thyroid health are generally dangerous or useless for thyroid disease patients, who may be purchasing them in the belief that it will restore thyroid function. Kelp, sargassum, and bladder wrack are especially noteworthy for these reasons. Manganese, iron, selenium (touted as "necessary for T4/T3 conversion"), magnesium, zinc, copper sulfur, and calcium are all sold as thyroid health supplements, but they do not have any effect on thyroid hormone conversion.

Goitrogens

Food substances and chemicals that interfere with the thyroid's production of thyroid hormone, often causing a goiter (an enlarged thyroid gland), are called *goitrogens*. In normal amounts by themselves, these goitrogens don't affect the thyroid; in regions of the world with iodine deficiency, however, these goitrogens worsen the incidence of hypothyroidism. One type of goitrogen, the thiocyanates, comes from foods such as yellow turnips, cassava, maize, bamboo shoots, sweet potatoes, and lima beans. Another type, the flavenoids, are found in millet, sorghum, beans, and ground nuts. Some goitrogens enter the water supply from coal deposits. Similarly, thiocyanates, flavenoids, and hydroxypyridines are goitrogenic chemicals that enter the body via cigarette smoke.

Known goitrogens include vegetables from the brassica family (cabbage, turnips, kohlrabi, bean sprouts, cauliflower) and cassava (tapioca). But unless your diet is severely iodine deficient, there is no need to worry about eating these foods, as they are excellent sources of fiber, important vitamins, and cancer-fighting agents.

Some lay people wonder whether large quantities of goitrogenic foods can cause hypothyroidism. Unfortunately, this is highly unlikely unless the diet is severely deficient in iodine and massive quantities of these raw foods are eaten. In the case of hyperthyroidism, such a diet could theoretically work to block the effects of thyroid hormone, but reality is not so obliging. It seems easier to take a methimazole tablet twice a day than to eat 20 pounds of raw cabbage, chew cassava, and follow a strict low-iodine diet each day. Also, a goitrogenic diet cannot cure the autoimmune disease that is causing thyrotoxicosis.

The Low-Iodine Diet

The typical amounts of stable iodine found in most diets can interfere with the use of radioactive iodine for the treatment of thyroid cancer. For radioactive iodine to work, it's important to starve the cancer cells of the relatively large quantities of nonradioactive iodine in your body so that the radioactive iodine is able to enter them. Your thyroid cancer cells can't tell the difference between radioactive iodine and stable, nonradioactive iodine. Stable iodine enters your body through your diet. A lot of dietary iodine comes from iodized salt. Additional iodine enters your diet from fish, seafood, kelp, dairy products, artificial red food dye (FD&C Red Dye #3), and multivitamins. If you follow a low-iodine diet prior to receiving radioactive iodine, your daily total iodine intake should be reduced from 500 mcg (the average daily intake) to less than 40 mcg, resulting in more than 12 times the amount of radio-activity being taken into each thyroid cancer cell than if you followed your usual diet. Thyroid cancer experts have noted over the years that patients on a low-iodine diet are frequently more responsive to scans (showing positive uptake) than those not on a low-iodine diet (often showing false negative uptake). Clearly, you don't want to have a false negative cancer screening, which means your scan does not show cancer when it is actually there.

A Brief History of the Low-Iodine Diet

Thyroid cancer specialists were aware of the value of a low-iodine diet for many years, although many of them could not agree on the composition of the diet. This became easier after a group at the National Institutes of Health (NIH) in Bethesda, Maryland, proposed a simple diet that proved to be effective. See Appendix B for suggested reading and additional resources to help you follow a low-iodine diet.

Low-Iodine Restrictions

Strict adherence to this diet will significantly enhance the sensitivity of the radioactive iodine scans and the effectiveness of any RAI treatments. The following foods or ingredients must be avoided on a low-iodine diet:

- Iodized salt, sea salt (noniodized salt may be used)
- Dairy products (milk, cheese, cream, yogurt, ice cream, butter)
- Eggs (specifically egg yolks; egg whites may be used)
- Seafood (both fresh and salt-water fish; shellfish; seaweed; kelp)
- Foods that contain the additives carrageenan, agar-agar, algin, or alginates

- Cured and corned foods (ham, corned beef, sausage, luncheon meats, sauerkraut, pickles)
- Bread products that contain iodate dough conditioners (breads from small bakeries are sometimes safe; better to bake it yourself from scratch)
- Foods and medications that contain red food dyes (specifically, FD&C Red Dye #3; consult your physician about discontinuing or substituting for any red-colored medicines)
- Chocolate (because of the milk content; dark or pareve chocolate is fine)
- Molasses
- Soy products (soy sauce, soy milk, tofu, soy burgers, etc.)

Additional Guidelines

- Avoid restaurant foods, since there's no reliable way to determine what's in your food.
- Use unsalted matzos (unleavened crackers made only of flour and water) or unsalted tortillas instead of bread.
- Noniodized salt may be used as desired.
- Read ingredient lists of prepared or packaged foods carefully.
- Do not take multivitamins, since most contain iodine.
- Use olive oil as a condiment or in cooking instead of butter or margarine; nondairy or pareve margarine may also be used.
- Prepare low-iodine meals in advance and freeze them for easy use later.
- Food prepared from any fresh meats, fresh poultry, fresh or frozen vegetables, and fresh fruits should be fine for this diet, provided that you do not add any of the "to avoid" ingredients listed. The diet is easiest when food is prepared from basic ingredients.

Inaccurate or Unproven Low-Iodine Diets

There are many versions of this diet that are inaccurate; some are very lax in that they tell patients to avoid only fish but that they can have everything else. The NIH recently modified the diet to allow some milk, although some insist that milk may completely spoil the diet and render it ineffective. Other patients and physicians have taken this diet to unnecessary extremes without proof that the excessiveness is necessary. Some claim that specific types of beans, rice, vegetables, or fruit should be avoided. Some versions of the diet propose that tap water and potato skins should be avoided.

One problem with these alternate diets is that many of the tables and assays for the iodine content of foods, beyond the stipulations of the basic low-iodine diet, are unreliable due to the difficulties in testing for iodine. Another problem is that a good low-iodine diet is not a no-iodine diet. The amount of iodine ingested in a twenty-four-hour period should be under 50 mcg. One way to assess this is to collect all the urine you produce in a twenty-four-hour period. The total amount of iodine in that urine sample reflects the total amount eaten during that time. In a variety of clinical trials, researchers measured the urine samples in many patients following the basic low-iodine diet and found it to be highly reliable without unnecessary additional restrictions.

Some thyroid cancer patient organizations, such as The Light of Life Foundation or ThyCa, offer downloadable recipes, but they are not kitchen tested. In the case of the ThyCa recipes, which many thyroid cancer patients use, the low-iodine diet used is the excessive one, banning certain types of rice and limiting quantities of meat and many types of vegetables. These excessive restrictions are unnecessary.

How Long to Follow a Low-Iodine Diet

You'll get different answers from different doctors regarding how long to stay on a low-iodine diet. Typical advice is to start the low-iodine diet two weeks before the radioactive iodine scan or treatment dose. For patients who are well versed on the diet, a week may be sufficient; however, most people make errors in the first week, thus requiring two weeks to reliably lower their stable iodine level. There is no advantage to spending longer periods of time on this diet prior to receiving radioactive iodine. Likewise, making significant errors on the diet just the day before receiving a radioactive iodine dose will

Shari's Story: My No-Fish Diet

When I needed to go on the low-iodine diet, I was being treated at a large, well-established hospital. I was given one simple instruction, which was hard for me as a vegetarian and someone with Celiac disease to follow: no fish. I was told I could have everything else, including milk and soy products. After I had my scan, I had some questions my doctor couldn't answer and I looked for a thyroid cancer expert elsewhere. When I found another doctor, he asked me if I had been on a low-iodine diet before my scan, and I said I had. I told him that it was no big deal, just not having fish, and he was shocked. He said that the scan was probably useless now and that I would have to do the whole thing again. When I went on the diet properly, the restrictions were much harder, as a lot of what I would normally eat as a vegetarian and "no flour child" were soy and dairy and fish. I found a few good recipes in the *Low Iodine Diet Cookbook* [see Appendix B] and lived off of the baking recipes, which I further adapted with gluten-free flour; vegetarian chili; fruit smoothies; and several of the salads and soups. Since I was also hypothyroid, I would not have been able to "think up" what to eat without having it written down. I'm used to adapting things anyway because of the gluten-free issue, but this was a real challenge.

undo all the good intentions of the entire two weeks on the low-iodine diet. There is no need to restrict your iodine intake for longer than twenty-four hours after swallowing a radioactive iodine treatment dose. This is because the entire effective uptake of radioactive iodine into thyroid cancer cells is finished by this time, making any further low-iodine dieting unnecessary. There is no need to prolong the low-iodine diet further, even if a posttherapy scan is performed at a later date. However, it may be necessary to continue the low-iodine diet for two or three days after taking the radioactive iodine scan dose, until all the diagnostic scans are completed and a decision is made regarding whether a radioactive iodine treatment dose is to be given. Nonetheless, once a decision has been made to not give a radioactive iodine treatment dose or twenty-four hours after the treatment dose has been given, there is no need to continue the low-iodine diet.

The Hypothyroid Diet for Life: Low Glycemic Index, Low Fat, and High Fiber

The best diet to follow if you are hypothyroid or euthyroid is a diet that combines the principles of most healthy diets today: a low–glycemic index diet (called low GI), as well as a high-fiber diet. These diets are heart healthy, colon friendly, and diabetes friendly and are naturally low in fat. The Weight Watchers core plan is essentially this type of diet.

There are several good low GI cookbooks available, as well as a myriad of sources about fiber. A high-fiber diet that is low in saturated fat and richer in unsaturated fat can help relieve constipation and bloat, fatigue, and weight gain. In essence, this is a diet for life that will help you feel better when you are combating periods of hypothyroidism because you're not properly balanced on thyroid hormone, as well as help to prevent cardiovascular and colon health problems. It will also compliment your thyroid medication, if you are balanced right now. And it will help you combat any preexisting weight problem that may be aggravated by your hypothyroidism.

The Glycemic Index

Low-glycemic eating, or the scientifically supported low-GI diet, emphasizes foods containing carbohydrates that break down slowly and thus release sugar into the bloodstream more slowly. These foods are called low glycemic index or low GI foods. The glycemic index ranks carbohydrate foods with a value of 0 to 100 according to their effect on blood sugar levels. Changes in blood sugar produced by a given food are measured against the rise in blood sugar produced by a load of sugar, or sucrose, which is 100 percent. To qualify as low GI, foods should have an index of 60 percent or less.

North America's obesity epidemic over the last three decades has coincided with an increased intake of carbohydrate-containing foods, many of which are high glycemic index. What has made matters worse is our tendency to eat one or two large meals a day. This results in tsunami-size insulin peaks, which predispose us to weight gain, as well as a host of symptoms and side effects that are a result of excess insulin in the blood. To address these symptoms and side effects, low GI eating calls for frequent, healthy low GI snacks to maintain steady low levels of insulin in the blood. This has been found to be a very beneficial diet for life, and it is also beneficial for thyroid patients— particularly those predisposed to Type 2 diabetes. Glycemic index food tables abound in books and online, and the information is pretty consistent in this area of health and nutrition. Stick to reliable nutrition or diet organization sites.

Increasing Fiber

Feeling bloated and constipated is a classic hypothyroid ailment. Much of the bloat is caused by constipation, as well as by not drinking enough water. What few people understand is that when you increase fiber, you have to increase your water intake as well. You can take fiber supplements and stool softeners while hypothyroid, which will help you when your fiber content is low. But these supplements can also be added to a high-fiber diet, discussed here. It's important to note that fiber supplements can interfere with the absorption of your thyroid hormone, so you should take them a few hours after your thyroid hormone, or try taking fiber at night and your thyroid hormone pill first thing in the morning.

Fiber is the part of a plant your body can't digest, which comes in the form of both water soluble fiber (dissolves in water) and water insoluble fiber (does not dissolve in water but, instead, absorbs water); this is what's meant by soluble and insoluble fiber. While soluble and insoluble fiber differ, they are equally beneficial.

Soluble fiber lowers the low-density lipid (LDL) cholesterol in your body. Experts aren't entirely sure how soluble fiber does this, but one popular theory is that it gets mixed into the bile the liver secretes and forms a type of gel that traps the building blocks of cholesterol, thus lowering your LDL levels.

Insoluble fiber doesn't affect your cholesterol levels at all, but it regulates your bowel movements. As the insoluble fiber moves through your digestive tract, it absorbs water like a sponge and helps to form your waste into a solid form more quickly, making the stools larger, softer, and easier to pass.

Good sources of soluble fiber include oats or oat bran, legumes (dried beans and peas), soybeans, some seeds, carrots, oranges, bananas, and other fruits.

Good sources of insoluble fiber are wheat bran and whole grains, skins from various fruits and vegetables, seeds, leafy greens, and cruciferous vegetables (cauliflower, broccoli, or Brussels sprouts).

Most of us will turn to grains and cereals to boost our fiber intake, which experts recommend should be at about 25–35 g per day. Aim for cereals that offer 5–10 g of fiber per serving. Double fiber breads offer 5 g of fiber per slice. One bowl of cereal; two slices of low-calorie, high-fiber bread; and some vegetable servings will get you to your 25–30 g per day. If you're a little under par, an easy way to boost your fiber intake is to simply take a fiber supplement or add pure wheat bran to your foods, which is available in health food stores or supermarkets. Three tablespoons of wheat bran is equal to 4.4 g of fiber.

Drinking Water with Fiber

It's important to drink water with fiber. Water means water. Milk, coffee, tea, soft drinks, and juice are not a substitute for water. Unless you drink water with your fiber, the fiber will not bulk up in your colon. Think of fiber as a sponge. Obviously, a dry sponge won't work; you must soak it with water for it to be useful. The same principle applies to fiber. In the general population, it's advised that you drink roughly 8 ounces of water with a fiber supplement. This is a good rule of thumb, but note that too much water can be dangerous when you're hypothyroid. Check with your doctor about how much water to drink with your fiber, as the amount will be based on your individual fiber intake and the extent to which you are hypothyroid.

Making Sense of Weight-Loss Diets

Dietary guidelines from nutrition experts, government nutrition advisories and panels, and registered dieticians have not changed in fifty years. A good diet is a balanced diet that represents all food groups; it should be grounded largely on plant-based foods, or carbohydrates, such as fruits, vegetables, legumes, and grains, with a balance of calories from animal-based foods, or proteins and fats, such as meats (red meat, poultry), fish, and dairy. Nutrition research spanning the last fifty years has only confirmed these facts. What has changed in fifty years is the terminology used to define a good diet and the bombardment of information we receive about which foods affect which physiological processes in the body, such as cholesterol levels, triglycerides, blood sugar levels, and insulin. There are also different kinds of fats and carbohydrates, which has made eating so technical and scientific that ordinary people feel more like chemists when trying to plan for healthy meals and diets.

No matter how many properties in foods are dissected or what kind of diet program you buy into, healthy eating comes down to a balanced diet—something that actually means "a balanced way of life." In fact, the root word of diet—*diatta*—literally means "way of life."

A diet is considered low fat when it restricts calories from fat to below 30 percent daily. There are dozens of established low-fat diets on the market, but they vary from extremely low-fat diets, which restrict calories from fat to about 10 percent, to more moderate low-fat diets, which restrict calories from fat to 15 to 30 percent. The limitations of the low-fat diet led people to gorge on "bad carbs" (meaning that they are high on the glycemic index, or considered simply sugars and starches) because they were led to believe that so long as a food was fat-free, it was healthy. Also, too few calories from fat left people hungry and craving food. Unfortunately, our society's habit of gorging on carbs has led to a sharp increase in insulin-resistance from carbohydrate overload in the diet.

Then came the diet backlash: the low-carb diet, the high-protein diet, or the Atkins diet. Low-carbohydrate diets are the opposite of low-fat diets: they restrict carbohydrates (which a healthy diet ought to be based on) to about 5 percent and encourage mostly high-fat foods—the more saturated fat, the better. In clinical circles, these diets are known as ketogenic diets because they trigger ketosis, a condition in which insulin production is shut down, forcing the liver to produce ketone bodies. The brain switches its nutritional status from using sugar as a primary fuel and starts to consume ketones. People can certainly lose weight while in ketosis, but living in a state of ketosis does not seem to be exactly what nature intended for a healthy human body. Hyperthyroidism tends to worsen ketosis, perhaps by decreasing the effect of insulin. In hypothyroidism, the liver function is impaired, possibly reducing the ability to safely tolerate a diet high in fat. Much is unknown concerning the metabolic interactions of an Atkins diet on people with thyroid disease.

In addition to the potential dangers of ketosis, the Atkins diet can cause terrible constipation in the first phase, badly aggravating the intestinal problems associated with hypothyroidism. In addition, consuming high levels of saturated fat spells disaster for people with hypothyroidism by exacerbating their cholesterol status, especially for those with high levels of LDL. Many people also have a genetic condition that causes high triglycerides, which cannot be controlled through diet alone; in these people, the Atkins diet can be life-threatening, causing pancreatitis (while a very low-fat diet has been shown, since the 1950s, to be life-saving). Other groups who are warned against the Atkins diet are those who suffer from any disease that puts a strain on the kidneys, such as hypertension, cardiovascular disease, and bladder infections or conditions. Of course, anyone who is pregnant should absolutely stay away from this diet.

Sound nutritional experts maintain that carbohydrates do not make us fat; it is overindulgence in carbohydrates or protein or fat that makes us fat. Eating fewer carbohydrates, less protein, and less fat—in other words, eating everything in moderation and expending more energy than is eaten—is the key to weight loss.

You can judge a good diet based on these four simple questions:

- Are all food groups present, including plant-based foods, grains, complex carbs, proteins, lean meats, and fats? If not, then stay away.
- Are you encouraged to take in the least number of calories from fats and discouraged from junk foods and refined sugars? If so, this is sensible.

- Is weight loss promised averaging about one to two pounds per week, or is weight loss promised of ten or more pounds a week? Anything more than one to two pounds a week is suspicious and likely faddish. Gradual weight loss is sustainable for life; speedy weight loss leads to yo-yo effects, in which you gain as much back as you lost and sometimes more.
- Is it a diet that offers enough variety that you would feel good eating this way for life? Is feeding your whole family with the foods encouraged? If not, be wary.

The Hyperthyroid Diet

If you are currently in the throes of hyperthyroidism and are thyrotoxic, it's important to note that your thyroid helps to control gastric emptying, secretion of digestive juices, and motility of the digestive tract. When you're thyrotoxic, despite a voracious appetite, you might lose weight and have hyperdefecation (frequent bowel movements). While thyrotoxic, increase your calcium intake by eating more butter, cream, cheese, and other dairy products. This will also help to keep your weight up. Peanut butter, mayonnaise, and animal fats can help as well. To reduce diarrhea, cut down on fruit juices and fresh fruits. Peanut butter is also good for binding. Sometimes, thyrotoxic people will develop sudden lactose intolerance, which can lead to gas and other unpleasantries. If this is the case, eliminate all milk products and take a calcium supplement while getting your fat from the other foods mentioned above.

Stay away from caffeine, alcohol, and cigarettes; all may stimulate your heart. You may want to take vitamin supplements as well. (Vitamins A, D, and E are stored in body fat and can be lost through excretion if you are thyrotoxic or hyperthyroid.) When you are in balance again, you will need to cut down on your fat and calcium intake.

Thyroid Disease and Obesity

Obesity refers to a body size that is too overweight for good health. Obese people have greater incidences of Type 2 diabetes, heart attacks, strokes, peripheral vascular disease (circulation problems, leading to many other health problems), and certain types of cancers. Hypothyroidism can aggravate obesity and complications caused by obesity. Hyperthyroidism or thyrotoxicosis may cause an unhealthy type of weight loss, exacerbating other conditions that may be linked to obesity, such as heart disease or Type 2 diabetes. It is not known how many people with thyroid disease are obese, but it is clear that the majority of obese people do not have thyroid disease. It is important to check for thyroid disease if you are obese, but you should not to be surprised when your thyroid tests are normal. There are many different causes of obesity. Nevertheless, many who are overweight may indeed be suffering from unrecognized or untreated hypothyroidism.

When obesity is due to hypothyroidism, most people will find that they start to return to their normal weight once their hypothyroidism is treated. Much of the weight gain in hypothyroidism is due to bloating. Of course, anything that causes you to gain additional body fat, such as pregnancy or hypothyroidism, may contribute to long-term obesity even after the cause is removed or treated. This is why you need to pay careful attention to diet and exercise even though you are taking the proper amount of thyroid hormone to have normal thyroid hormone levels and a normal TSH level.

Feelings of tiredness and low energy, which are symptoms of hypothyroidism, may cause you to crave carbohydrates and quick-energy foods, which are higher in fat and calories. When you are hypothyroid, your activity levels will decrease as a result of your fatigue, which can also lead to weight gain or aggravate preexisting obesity. The craving for carbohydrates is caused by a desire for energy. Consuming carbohydrates produces an initial rush of energy, but that rush is soon followed by a "crash," sometimes known as *postprandial depression* (or *postmeal depression*), exacerbating or contributing to *hypothyroid-induced depression*. Even in people with normal thyroid function, depression can cause cravings for simple carbohydrates such as sugars and sweets. In the absence of overeating, some of the weight gain in hypothyroidism is generally bloating caused by constipation.

A problem for many people who are battling both obesity and hypothyroidism is that their obesity often predates their thyroid problem, indicating that there were other factors involved in their weight gain. Stack a thyroid problem on top of that, and it may aggrieve other behaviors that led to the initial weight gain, as well as aggravate risks associated with obesity in general.

Defining Obesity

Obesity is best defined by the Body Mass Index (BMI). The BMI is calculated by dividing your weight (in kilograms) by your height (in meters) squared. (The formula used is: BMI = kg/m^2 if you're doing this on your calculator.) BMI charts abound on websites, on the backs of cereal boxes, and in numerous health magazines. Most people can now easily find BMI converters on the Internet, where you simply type in your weight in pounds and your height to arrive at your BMI. A good chart will calculate BMI by gender and sometimes even age ranges.

Currently, a BMI of 18.5 or less indicates that you are underweight. A BMI of between 18.5 and 24.9 is normal. The most recent clinical guidelines define people with a BMI of between 25 and 29.9 as over-weight, and those with a BMI of between 30 and 34.9 as obese (mild to moderate). A BMI of between 35.0 and 39.9 indicates severe obesity; people with a BMI of 40 or greater are considered morbidly obese.

Waist circumference is another factor in calculating obesity, par-ticularly abdominal obesity. Men with a waist circumference of 40 inches or more and women with a waist circumference of 35 inches or more are at increased risk of obesity-related health problems.

North Americans have the highest obesity rates in the world. More than half of North American adults and about 25 percent of North American children are now overweight or obese. These figures reflect a doubling of adult obesity rates since the 1960s and a dou-bling of the childhood obesity rate since the late 1970s—a stagger-ing increase when you think about it in raw numbers. According to the most recent research, obese children will most likely grow up to become obese adults.

Biological Causes of Obesity

The physiological cause of obesity is eating more calories than you burn. People gain weight for two reasons: they may eat excessively (often excessive amounts of nutritious foods), which results in daily consumption of too many calories, or they may eat moderately but simply be too inactive to burn the calories they do ingest.

Obesity experts consider lifestyle to be the single largest contributing factor to obesity. Although social, behavioral, metabolic, cellular, and genetic factors all contribute to obesity, some obesity genes are turned on only in the presence of a lifestyle conducive to weight gain, such as a sedentary and food-rich lifestyle. Genetic makeup can predispose some body types to obesity earlier in life. Experts in nutrition agree that genetics plays only a small role in the sharp increase in obesity. Since genetic changes take place over centuries, and our obesity rate has at least doubled since the 1960s, it's fairly obvious that lifestyle factors are the chief culprit. Furthermore, as we age, our metabolism slows down. This means that unless we decrease our calories or increase activity levels to compensate, we will probably gain weight.

Obesity is a complex problem. By most accounts, obesity is caused by a toxic environment: sedentary living, too much cheap or convenient food (a problem known as the "diet of poverty"), and not enough exercise naturally engineered into our lifestyle. Chapter 12 discusses the critical role of exercise as a complementary activity for thyroid patients, and it obviously can help combat obesity as well.

The typical obese person with thyroid disease frequently has multiple problems going on at once; these are usually complications of obesity that can become magnified with thyroid disease. For example, many obese people with thyroid disease are also managing high cholesterol, hypertension, and Type 2 diabetes. Worse, a number of these people are also smokers, which aggravates preexisting obesity complications and current diagnoses. It's a complex health care puzzle for most thyroid specialists.

The key to managing thyroid disease in obese people is to treat all problems at once: the thyroid problem *and* the obesity *and* all other health complications. This is rare. Many physicians only treat one complication at a time and don't get anywhere. Thyroid specialists know to jump right in. It's not unusual for a thyroid doctor to initiate prescriptions for thyroid hormone, cholesterol- and blood pressure–lowering medications, and the most important prescription: a healthy diet for weight loss at the same time. Restoring thyroid function to the obese individual may not contribute so much to a feeling of overall health unless weight loss also occurs.

12

Complementary Activities and Therapies

When You Need a Massage

THIS CHAPTER IS about evidence-based complementary activities and therapies for thyroid patients. This chapter will give you solid information about what works to reduce stress, depression, and anxiety; to improve your quality of life and sense of well-being; and to combat low energy and weight gain.

Becoming Active

The most common complaints among posttreatment thyroid patients are weight gain, bloating and constipation, and fatigue. If your TSH level is normal and you are euthyroid, the most common reason for these symptoms is lack of exercise. In fact, one of the most overlooked complementary activities for thyroid disease is exercise. The evidence has been mounting for years, but once you hit your forties and fifties, you can no longer retain your shape and energy levels without incorporating some exercise, even if you are dieting.

Exercise creates endorphins, which are hormones that make you feel good. It also works your body and heart muscles and helps to relieve many of the symptoms attributed to hypothyroidism, including constipation. Aerobic activities increase oxygen flow, which helps burn fat. Your breathing improves, your blood pressure improves, and your heart works better. More oxygen also makes your brain work better, so you feel better. In addition, oxygen lowers triglycerides and cholesterol, increasing high-density lipoproteins (HDL), the good cholesterol, while decreasing low-density lipoproteins (LDL), the bad cholesterol. In addition to the usual machines at the gym, activities such as cross-country skiing, walking, hiking, and biking are all aerobic. Dancing can also be an aerobic activity, depending on the type. Find something you like doing, and do it one to three times per week for ten minutes. As the activity gets easier, increase your time by five minutes until you can do it for thirty minutes one to three times per week.

Active Living

Many people become sedentary over time due to too much driving, sedentary jobs, and so forth. If it's too difficult to start regular exercise, health promotion experts advise active living as the first step in becoming unsedentary. There are many ways you can adopt an active lifestyle. Here are some suggestions:

- If you drive everywhere, pick the parking space farthest away from your destination so you can work some daily walking into your life.
- If you take public transit everywhere, get off one or two stops early so you can walk the rest of the way to your destination.
- Choose the stairs over the escalators and elevators.
- Park at one side of the mall and then walk to the other.
- Stroll around your neighborhood after dinner.
- Get a dog, as you'll need to walk it.
- On weekends, go to the zoo or to flea markets, garage sales, and other venues where you need to walk.
- Consider a lower-impact weekly activity, such as ballroom dancing, belly dancing, swimming, and so on.

Stretching

Stretching improves muscle blood flow, oxygen flow, and digestion. The natural desire to stretch is there for those reasons. The follow-

Elana's Story: HypoTango

I found it difficult to feel like myself again after I was treated for Hashimoto's disease. I kept going in for TSH tests and my doctor kept telling me it was normal, reminding me that there are other things that can make me feel tired and gain weight, and telling me that all his patients complain about it who have normal thyroids, too. He also reminded me that before I had become hypo, I was hyperthyroid from Hashitoxicosis. I was about thirty-six when my Hashimoto's disease was diagnosed, and I found that by thirty-nine, I just couldn't seem to keep the weight off. I didn't know if it was my thyroid, or my age, or what. I got very down and sort of cocooned for a few months. I think I was depressed. My girlfriend bought me a fortieth birthday present of free ballroom dancing lessons. I *really* didn't want to do it, but she went with me. I started to really like it, and the music, and the people just helped to make me feel alive again. I learned the tango and got pretty good at it. I bought myself another ten weeks of lessons and just kept going. They would have dances every Friday night for all of the ex-students to practice with each other. I met a lot of people, and eventually, some of the weight started to come off.

ing stretches will help relieve tension, muscular aches and pains, and fatigue and will improve your overall sense of well-being.

- While sitting or standing, raise your arms above your head. Keep your shoulders relaxed and breathe deeply for five seconds. Release and repeat five times.
- Gently raise your shoulders in an exaggerated shrug. Breathe deeply and hold for ten seconds. Relax and repeat three times.
- Sit on your heels. Bring your forehead to the floor in front of you. Breathe into the back of your ribcage, feeling the stretch in your spine. Hold for as long as it's comfortable.

- Stand tall and find a point across the room on which to focus your gaze. Place the heel of one foot on the opposite inner thigh. Float your arms upward until your palms are touching. Breathe deeply and hold for five seconds. Release and repeat on the other side.
- Lie on your back with your palms facing upward, your feet turned gently outward. Focus on the movement of breath throughout your body.

Yoga

Yoga is designed to tone and soothe your mental and physical state. Most people benefit from introductory yoga classes or even introductory yoga videos, and almost every health club or gym these days offers a yoga class. Yoga does a few things for people with thyroid disease:

- Aids with toning and weight loss. Many of the postures work your core muscle group, which helps with abdominal weight in particular.
- Aids with improving oxygen flow throughout the body (through the yogic breath), which relieves fatigue, improves a sense of well-being, and can reduce stress and other risk factors for hypertension.
- Aids with muscular aches and pains that are aggravated by hypothyroidism.
- Aids anxiety and restlessness that are aggravated by thyrotoxicosis.

Qigong

Every morning, all over China, people of all ages gather at parks to do their daily qigong exercises. The word *qi* means vitality, energy, and life force; the word *gong* means practice, cultivate, and refine. Pronounced "ch'i kung," these exercises work on the principle of "life force energy," helping it to flow or unblock. No one really knows if this energy, or *qi*, exists, but there are many benefits to qigong exercises. The exercises have a continuous flow, rather than the stillness of a posture seen in yoga, and they are modeled after movements in wildlife, such as birds or animals, of trees, and of other things in nature.

Using the hands in various positions to gather in the qi, move the qi, or release the qi is one of the most important aspects of qigong movements. These exercises look more like a dance with precise, slow movements; they are similar to tai chi, except they allow for greater flexibility in routine.

The Chinese believe that practicing qigong balances the body and improves physical and mental well-being. These exercises are meant to push the life-force energy into the various meridian pathways that correspond to organs, incorporating the same map used in pressure point therapies. Qigong improves oxygen flow and enhances the lymphatic system.

The best place to learn qigong is through a qualified instructor, rather than from a book or video. You can generally find qigong classes through the alternative healing community, but many local health clubs offer classes these days. Check health food stores and other centers that offer classes such as yoga or tai chi.

For Your Mental Health

Living with thyroid disease can tax your mental health in a variety of ways. If you are like many thyroid patients, getting an accurate diagnosis can take a long time. In addition, getting to a balanced, euthyroid state can take time, particularly if you have Graves' disease or thyroid cancer. Bouts of hypothyroidism or thyrotoxicosis can wreak havoc on your life and affect your work and social network. The thread that keeps us all mentally fit and healthy is fine; when we load chronic illness, fear of the unknown, and the myriad extra stresses that feeling unwell can create, the thread can break. Here are some tips from mental health experts that can help you regain a sense of self if you feel you've lost your center or feel you are suffering from depression.

Stay Socially Connected

The large body of work that looks at causes of stress, sadness, and depression shows us that people suffer most when they are feeling disconnected from the world around them. When we feel plugged in to our community and network of friends and colleagues, it brings us increased zest, well-being, and motivation. Connection brings us increased self-worth, as well as a desire to make more connections.

Cutting ourselves off from people can also cause loneliness. Loneliness is stressful; solitude is rejuvenating. Loneliness comes from a lack of truly intimate relationships with friends or family members; intimacy, in this case, refers to sharing deep feelings, fears, and so on with someone. This is how we unburden ourselves and relieve stress. Feeling as though you belong somewhere or feeling like part of a community can also alleviate loneliness. This is one reason why faith-based activities have seen such a revival in the last decade; the more we technologize our world, the more people seek a basic sense of community again.

Here are steps you can take to create more supportive relationships in your life or to develop more of a sense of community:

• Thyroid online support can be blessing and a curse, depending on who you meet online and on what you're reading, but you will certainly meet people who are going through what you're going through. Finding support solely online can breed social isolation as you become dependent on the computer and not on live people. If you meet people online, try to organize live meetings or support groups or to look for someone nearby who you can meet for lunch.

• If you are a person of faith or are seeking those who share the same cultural values, you can contact cultural centers or churches/synagogues/mosques for information about community, faith-based, or cultural activities.

• Find some sort of social group to belong to by looking into gourmet cooking clubs, art classes, and so on. Find an activity that you're really drawn to; chances are you'll meet like-minded souls with whom you can form quality friendships.

• Have a couple of nice dinner parties each year. It's a way to create more intimate friendships with people who may be only acquaintances or casual friends.

• Get involved in your neighborhood or community. Whether it's a "not in my backyard" lobby or a community street sale, get out and meet your neighbors. Responding to community-based programs, parents/kids activities, bake sales, sports events, and so forth is the way to find support. In fact, community outreach workers actually use arts, crafts, fitness, and computer classes as a tool to attract people within the community who could benefit from support. What often takes place in community-based programs is a great deal of talking and sharing prior to, during, or after the activity. These are places where you make friends, find someone you can talk to, and, most importantly, find that you're not alone.

• Volunteering for causes dear to your heart is a great way to meet people and to feel needed. In fact, many thyroid organizations run on volunteers who have been through what you have. Other common places to volunteer include meals on wheels programs, eldercare facilities, street youth programs, and so forth; all attract wonderful souls with whom you may find friendship and comfort.

• Getting a dog is not only a great physical activity, it's also great for staying connected. Dogs need to be walked, which means you'll meet other people walking their dogs. And dog owners tend to gravitate toward other dog owners. It's a great jumping-off point for meeting people. Aside from that, many studies point to the health effects of pet ownership, including lowered blood pressure and lowered incidences of heart disease. (Positive health effects can be seen with any pet, including cats.)

Eliminate Energy Drains

Many thyroid patients find that their bouts with hypothyroidism, thyrotoxicosis, or thyroid cancer expose something they may not have noticed before: energy drains.

Most energy drains come in the form of people. While you may have had the mental energy for draining people in the past, after dealing with a health problem, you may discover that you need to shake off people who don't help you. When you're surrounded by people who take energy from you, rather than give you energy in the form of support, the result is less energy, more stress in your life, and more difficulty managing illness. By doing a serious reevaluation of your personal relationships, you may be able to find more energy and reduce the amount of stress in your life. Ask yourself some of the following questions:

• Do you have someone in your life who offers judgment-free emotional support? This means a person who makes you feel positive about yourself rather than a person who points out your flaws or attacks your choices.

- Are there people in your life who drain your energy and reserves? These are people who always seem to be in crisis and suck up large amounts of "free therapy" time from you, but they never seem to be there for you. These can also be people who criticize you and make you feel negative and hopeless instead of positive and optimistic.
- Do you have unresolved conflicts with family members or friends? These unresolved feelings can drain your energy and focus when you obsess about the conflict.
- Do you feel that your friends are more like acquaintances and that you lack truly intimate friendships?
- Do you feel a void in your life because there is an absence of a romantic partner?
- Are you in a romantic or sexual relationship that you need to end, but you have been avoiding doing so?
- Are you in a relationship that compromises your values?
- Is there a phone call you need to make but are avoiding, which is causing you stress and anxiety?
- Is there someone in your life who continuously breaks commitments or plans, with whom you are constantly rescheduling?

Energy drains can also come from unmet needs in your home environment. Do you have broken appliances, car repairs that haven't been done, a wardrobe you hate, cluttered closets and rooms, or even ugly surroundings? Living in a home that is not decorated in a way that pleases you makes you feel as though you don't want to be there. Plants, paint, covers for ugly furniture, and a few things on the wall often make the difference between barren and cozy surroundings.

Finally, energy drains come from procrastinating and overbooking yourself. You may have a tendency to procrastinate over things you really don't want to do, such as taxes. You may overbook yourself when you're afraid of saying no. Simply doing too much and expecting too much from yourself can drain your energy. When possible, hire someone to do the things you can't or don't want to do. You can hire people to:

- Clean your house or apartment
- Declutter your house by going through closets, drawers, and stacks of papers, and start filing things

- Organize your tax receipts
- Take care of your garden and/or lawn

Counseling and Talk Therapy

The most overlooked complementary therapy for thyroid disease is talk therapy. What may be causing you stress, anxiety, and depression once your thyroid problems are treated often has nothing to do with your thyroid—or lack thereof—and more to do with other things going on in your life.

From time to time, one of the best things you can do is to talk to a professional—especially when you feel your life has been turned upside down by an unexpected illness or health problem. Simply finding someone objective to talk to can make an enormous difference. Most people looking for "sorting out your life" counseling do well with counselors or social workers, but the following professionals can all help:

- **Psychologist and Psychological Associate.** This is someone who can be licensed to practice therapy with either a master's or a doctoral degree. Clinical psychologists have a master of science degree (M.Sc.) or master of arts (M.A.); they can also hold a doctor of philosophy (Ph.D.) in psychology, a doctor of education (Ed.D.), or a doctor of psychology (Psy.D.). They will usually work in a hospital or clinic setting but often can be found in private practice.
- **Social Worker.** This professional holds a bachelor of social work (B.S.W.) and/or a master of social work (M.S.W.) degree; some social workers have doctor of social work (D.S.W.) degrees as well. A professional social worker has a degree in social work and meets state legal requirements. The designation C.S.W. stands for certified social worker and is a legal title granted by the state. A designation of A.C.S.W. refers to a national credential granted by the nongovernmental organization the National Association of Social Workers and stands for the Academy of Certified Social Workers. The C.S.W. requires graduation (in most states) from a master's level program as well as passing an exam, while the ACSW requires an additional two years of supervised experience following graduation from such a program. Some social workers have a P or an R, which indicate C.S.W.s who have become qualified under state law to receive insurance reim-

Angela's Story: Cleanliness Was Next to Euthyroidism

I was diagnosed with Hashimoto's disease after I had my third baby, and I had little ones at home. My husband was working two jobs and was never home anymore. I sort of lost it after the thyroid problem; I just felt like a robot with the children and let a lot of things go. The house became a mirror image of my brain: disorganized, messy, and no order to anything. My TSH tests were showing that my thyroid was balanced (the readings were about 2.0). But I kept questioning my readings and wondering why I was feeling so crappy. My doctor sat me down one day and said: "Look—you have two toddlers, a newborn, and no help. *Anyone* would feel 'hypothyroid' under these circumstances." I just started to cry, and I had to go into the waiting room to collect myself. Another patient who was waiting had really terrible, bulging eyes, and she asked me, "Thyroid trouble?" I just started to cry again and told her that my tests were fine, but I couldn't get it together. She asked me how many kids I had and then gave me her card—she ran a corporate cleaning company and said, "All this stress has blown out my thyroid gland, so I've hired more girls. You can be my first residence; I want to train some girls to clean houses. What if we came tomorrow and did a freebie and counted it as training?" I took her up on it. They came and cleaned my house: they sorted my laundry, changed my linens, and got the kitchen looking organized. I felt like a new person. It made the biggest difference. The toilets were the best part. I hired this company to come once a month and get my house together. It just made me feel like I could handle the other parts of my life again.

bursement for outpatient services to clients with group health insurance. Each initial refers to different types of insurance policies: the P requires three years of supervised experience, while the R requires six years.

- **Psychiatric Nurse.** A psychiatric nurse is most likely a registered nurse (R.N.) with a bachelor of science in nursing (B.Sc.), although this isn't absolutely required. He or she probably has a master's degree in nursing, too, which could be either a master of arts (M.A.) or a master of science (M.Sc.). But whatever the degree, this nurse has done most of his or her training in a psychiatric setting and may also be trained to do psychotherapy.
- **Counselor.** Counselors have usually completed certification courses in counseling and therefore have obtained a license to practice psychotherapy; they may have, but do not require, a university degree. Counselors will frequently have a master's degree in a related field, such as social work, or they may have a master's degree in a field having nothing to do with mental health. The term *professional counselor* is used to represent those persons who have earned a minimum of a master's degree and possess professional knowledge and demonstrable skills in the application of mental health, psychological, and human development principles to facilitate human development and adjustment throughout the life span. Most states have enacted some type of counselor credentialing law that regulates the use of titles related to the counseling profession. The letters *CPC* stand for certified professional counselor, which refers to the title granted by the state legislative process. The letters *LPC* stand for licensed professional counselor, the most-often-granted state statutory counselor credential. No matter what letters you see, however, it's always a good idea to ask your counselor what training he or she has had in the field of mental health.
- **Marriage and Family Counselor.** This is somewhat different than the broader term *counselor*. This professional has completed rigorous training through certification courses in family therapy and relationship dynamics and has obtained a license to practice psychotherapy. This professional should have the designation MFT. MFTs have graduate training (a master's or doctoral degree) in marriage and family therapy and at least two years of clinical experience. Forty-one states currently license, certify, or regulate MFTs.

Feel-Good Therapies That Work!

The following complementary therapies both feel good and work.

Massage

Massage therapy can be beneficial whether you're receiving the massage from your spouse or a massage therapist trained in any one of dozens of techniques from shiatsu to Swedish massage. If you're hypothyroid, massage therapy may help to improve circulation and depression; if you're thyrotoxic, it can help to relieve anxiety and calm you down. In Chinese medicine, massage is recommended as

Anya's Story: "Tell Me About Your Thyroid"

I made an appointment with a therapist because I just couldn't stop obsessing about my health after I was treated for thyroid cancer. I used to feel sure of myself and in control, and after my thyroid cancer, I just didn't trust my body and started to have a lot of anxiety. I went to see someone that worked with a lot of cancer patients, and she asked me to talk to her first about my thyroid and what it meant to me. One of the things she pointed out was that it was a part of me I never really thought about much before—but a part that made everything "work." So I guess I lost something I never knew I had until I lost it. I had taken it for granted. Now it was gone. She recommended that I start to really grieve about losing my thyroid, and we spent a few sessions talking about grief—for a thyroid gland of all things! But it was a part of myself that I lost, and it was important to me. She encouraged me to find something that would honor the loss, and I bought a butterfly necklace. I wear it as a surrogate thyroid gland now, and, although it seems silly, I guess I just needed to acknowledge that I was sad about it. It turns out there were a whole bunch of other things I was taking for granted in my life that I started to pay more attention to. The therapy continued for about a year, but I realized that it wasn't just about thyroid cancer—it was more like the cancer exposed something I wasn't ready to look at, and now I can.

a treatment for a variety of illnesses; tuina massage, a form of deep tissue massage, combined with acupuncture is very effective. A Swedish doctor and poet, Per Henrik, borrowed techniques from ancient Egypt, China, and Rome to develop Swedish massage (what most of us Westerners are familiar with) in the nineteenth century. It's out of shiatsu in the East and Swedish massage in the West that the many forms of massage were developed.

Types of massage include:

- Deep tissue massage
- Manual lymph drainage
- Neuromuscular massage
- Sports massage
- Swedish massage
- Shiatsu massage

See Appendix B for some resources that explain these types of massage in detail.

Massage relaxes muscles to improve blood flow throughout connective tissues; it is more technically referred to as soft tissue manipulation. But no matter what kind of massage you have, there exist numerous, helpful gliding and kneading techniques used along with deep circular movements and vibrations that will relax muscles, improve circulation, and increase mobility. All are known to help relieve stress, which can be aggravated if you're in the middle of treatment for thyroid disease or can be due to other lifestyle factors. It also can ease muscle and joint pain, which frequently heightened by bouts of hypothyroidism. In people undergoing treatment for thyroid cancer, massage can help to ease stress, as well as help cancer patients stay grounded or centered while going through the balancing act of thyroid hormone replacement. Some established benefits of massage include:

- Improved circulation
- Improved lymphatic system
- Faster recovery from musculoskeletal injuries
- Soothed aches and pains
- Reduced edema (water retention)
- Reduced anxiety

Massage is so beneficial to a person's sense of well-being that a number of employers cover massage therapy in their health plans.

Acupuncture

Acupuncture is also called a pressure point therapy; it is an ancient Chinese healing art that aims to restore the smooth flow of what the Chinese call "life force energy" (qi) to the body. While no one has established whether the qi exists, it doesn't really matter, because well-done studies have shown that there are proven benefits to acupuncture. There are close to thirteen thousand peer-reviewed journal articles acknowledging the benefits of acupuncture.

Acupuncturists believe that your qi can be accessed from various points on your body, such as your ear. Each point is associated with a specific organ, and each of the roughly two thousand points on your body has a specific therapeutic effect when stimulated. Depending on your physical health, an acupuncturist will use a fine needle on a very specific point to restore qi to various organs. Acupuncture can relieve many of the physical symptoms and ailments caused by stress; it's now believed by most allopathic, or conventional, physicians that acupuncture stimulates the release of endorphins, which is why it's effective in reducing stress, anxiety, and pain.

Meditation

Meditation can be either an activity or a therapy. Meditation helps you relax. Particularly important if you're anxious about your thyroid treatments or if you're thyrotoxic, meditation simply requires you to stop thinking (about your life and your problems) and just be. Yogic breathing is a tool for meditation often used to get you to focus solely on your breath. Breathing deeply in through one nostril and out through your mouth is the classic technique. To do this, people usually find a relaxing spot, sit quietly, and breathe deeply for a few minutes.

There is also active meditation, which can include:

- Walking or hiking
- Swimming

- Running or jogging
- Gardening
- Playing golf
- Listening to music
- Dancing
- Reading for pleasure
- Walking your dog
- Practicing breathing exercises—or simply listening to the sounds of your own breathing
- Practicing stretching exercises
- Practicing yoga or qigong

Be Informed: Complementary and Alternative Therapies

It's important to note that there is a difference between complementary therapies and alternative therapies. Complementary therapies are those that work along with, or complement, allopathic (conventional) treatments. Alternative therapies take the place of allopathic treatments. But be careful: alternative therapies are often unproven, meaning that they may either have no proven benefit or may even be potentially harmful. The term *alternative* is misleading because it is not really an alternative when you're choosing between a proven therapy and an unproven therapy. Complementary therapies, however, demonstrate reasonable evidence that the activity or therapy may complement your allopathic therapies for thyroid treatment—or, at the very worst, that they will do no harm. All therapies described in this chapter are considered complementary.

Appendix A

How to Assess Thyroid Books, Websites, and Other Resources

WHEN YOU'RE NAVIGATING the Internet or looking for other accessible literature on thyroid disease, it's hard to tell whether what you're reading is accurate. The purpose of this appendix is to teach you how to apply critical thinking skills to the health information you're accessing. It is up to each author or website owner's discretion whether to circulate content for peer review or medical review. Even then, the information may not be completely consistent or accurate, since there are different opinions within the medical community.

Navigating Academic Journal Articles: The Problem

Many people look for health information by doing their own searches of the peer-reviewed medical journal literature on PubMed. This sounds like a great idea, but it creates additional problems. If you do not have a medical background or have no formal training (meaning graduate-level training) in science or medicine, the medical literature is wide open for misinterpretation. There are thousands of publications people can look through, but some are based on poor studies, while others are based on good studies. Some are bad review articles, some are good review articles. Conflicts of interest and bias are other problems that can pollute the literature. It is difficult enough for scientists and doctors to sift through the literature and use it effectively; it is simply not possible for a layperson without some training in science or medicine to do the same. Many patient advocacy websites now offer opinions or "translations" of medical literature for the lay browser. The result can be disastrous: a misinterpreted article can travel through listserves and websites like a virus. That's how misinformation occurs. There is no real solution to the problem of eliminating the wide gaps in knowledge between the "medical science education" haves and have nots.

Guidelines for Searching the Medical Literature

When searching the Internet for medical information, start with links from credible sources (see Appendix B), which are accountable to the public trust. They will do a reasonable job of boiling down the facts. Stay clear of individual patient sites or blogger sites. And make sure to refer to the critical thinking skills section below. If you're doing a PubMed search, visit a public library and discuss with the librarian how to look for review articles. A review article summarizes how the condition/disease you're interested in was once viewed and treated by the medical community and takes it to where we are today, as of the publication date of the article. These types of articles are a little easier to follow. You will not be able to determine whether it is a good or bad review article, which often has a lot to do with familiarity of the academic players and authors involved in the review. This is not meant as an insult; you just *can't* know that unless you work in the field. Stay clear of articles that report on laboratory studies, also known as bench research: these have no relevance to what happens in the clinical arena. And if they do, you won't understand how unless you can boast credentials in one of the basic sciences, such as molecular biology or microbiology. Even then, scientific disciplines are very specific. Some journals are referenced journals, but not peer-reviewed; these may contain summary articles that are easier to follow, but the articles have not been peer-reviewed and could still be biased.

What Is a Credible Source of Information Online?

Credible sources of information online are generally professional associations accountable to the public trust; professionals accountable to the public trust who must adhere to ethical guidelines within their professions; or recognized charitable organizations (who must have a medical advisory board) that are appropriately registered as charities, which are also accountable to the public trust. This does not mean that all information on such websites is completely up to date or accurate, since there is often wide disagreement within the medical community about various issues. But it reasonably ensures that blatant spin or fabrication does not occur on these websites.

Critical Thinking Skills: How to Apply Them

If you've seen the film *The Wizard of Oz*, you'll remember that finding out who the man is behind the curtain is a good example of critical thinking skills. In this case, you'll need to find out who the person is behind the information you're reading. The following are a few important questions to answer before spending your time reading anything.

• What is the copyright date of the material? Is it current? Health content offering prescriptive advice that is more than than five years old is usually substantially out of date. Descriptions of biological processes can even change as new understanding of various conditions becomes available, but it depends on the topic. For content that involves a review of the literature, known as a review article (summary articles that look at "where have we been, where are we going"), older materials are very relevant. Material that discusses sociological, ethical, or other theoretical concepts does not date and can remain relevant for decades. Material that discusses law and policy may be relevant for decades, depending on the topic.
• What is the education, background, and training of the author? Authors or journalists with no specific medical credentials are cred-

ible, so long as their content is put through a medical review. Authors with doctorates, who write about health content, can be medical social scientists, medical historians, or basic science researchers. (I am a bioethicist and medical sociologist.) Of course training is very important too. Sometimes the author with a Ph.D. has been through more rigorous training in academic critical literature and is better situated to judge references and resources than physicians who have had no training in academic medical research. Note, however, that some people who claim to have a Ph.D. received it through a nonaccredited institution or through a sham operation online. That means they do not have a recognized doctorate but have used the credential on their materials to fool the public into thinking they have more education than they do. Physician authors may be biased if the content has not been peer-reviewed, but they are also more likely to have had a ghostwriter, which means that the content was generated by a professional writer who then had the doctor vet it for accuracy. In these cases, the doctor is the "author" of the book or website for contractual purposes, but he or she has really played the role of medical editor.

• Do you even know who the author is? If no one claims ownership over text you find online, its credibility is highly suspect.

• How does the author or website profit from the information provided? For example, the health "Guides" on About.com get paid by the "hit," which would suggest that content has been sensationalized to draw in browsers. Some websites are completely sponsored by pharmaceutical companies, although in many cases the medical content is still accurate, since such companies have medical advisors on staff.

• Does the author promote products, or do advertisements accompany the material? Does the author/blogger promote particular herbs, supplements, or brand-name products? Such promotion could be suspect unless these products are standard of care.

• Does the author disclose all potential conflicts of interest? Disclosing the potential conflict means the conflict has been ethically managed. Once the author discloses the conflict, the public can make an assessment as to whether the work was influenced, and the work is therefore open to public debate and scrutiny.

• Does the content make sweeping generalizations without proper references?

- Does the author editorialize, offering just his or her opinion, or is the article an informed review, citing relevant literature?
- Does the content make potentially defamatory statements about someone? Personal attacks are a sign that the author is very unprofessional and lacks credibility. People who can't formulate intelligent arguments resort to name calling and discrediting.

Is the Content Put Through a Medical Review?

A medical review means that an author with no formal medical training submits content he or she generates to one or two medical experts in the field for editing and corrections. (I have done this with all my books.) A medical advisor is preferably an expert in the topic, rather than a generalist with no specific recognition in the field or topic in question. This may mean the advisor is a nutritionist or is specially credentialed in a certain medical technology. The more specific the medical content, the more specially trained the medical advisor ought to be. When you see a health website or a book written by someone with no formal medical training, find out if the content has been reviewed by someone with relevant medical credentials. Acknowledgments or forewords will often reveal who the expert reviewers were. If a website is just a free-for-all blogger environment, the website may be entertaining, but it is probably full of inaccuracies.

Content that does not need a medical review is health narrative. Content that does need a medical review is content that describes health conditions and offers information on symptoms, treatment options, and specific research in that area. Reviews of peer-reviewed academic medical literature also need a medical review.

What Is Health Narrative?

A health narrative is literature in which the health content being offered is clearly subjective and relates the experience of one or many individuals. This is an important type of health knowledge to share, as it validates others' health experiences. Health authors such as patients or bloggers who state that the content is their story need to be read within the appropriate context of a storyteller, and these texts should not be construed as prescriptive advice about a disease. Some websites or books mix narrative with advice. Many websites begin as narrative and expand into advice, without adding medical review to the advice portion of their text. All listserves should be considered health narrative. Many listserves have a medical advisor monitoring the content to ensure that narrative doesn't cross the line into advice; such advisors may jump in and send posts that correct potentially dangerous misinformation.

Internet health browsers who don't understand the difference between narrative and advice often base their decision making on the subjective narratives they read, which may also quote from other sources (usually misconstrued as well). When you read, "I had a bad reaction to drug X," it is narrative. When you read, "I read in journal X that herb Y cures disease X," it is narrative. In the case of this book, I use patients' stories to validate the information I provide, not the other way around.

What Does Peer-Reviewed Literature Mean?

Peer review means that content generated by someone trained in a special area is circulated to his or her academic or medical peers, who are similarly trained in a similar area, so they can comment on the content; point out errors, bias, or distortions; or suggest improvements. That makes for more objective, accurate content. For example, all academic journals are peer-reviewed. When academic articles are written, the author submits his or her article to the journal. The journal circulates it to three or four academic peers, or experts in the topic the author is writing about. These peers critically assess the content and make recommendations as to whether it's good enough to be published. Many publications submitted to journals are rejected; many are revised and resubmitted for reconsideration. This process helps to create content that is reasonably accurate and unbiased. It's not a perfect process, but it's the best checks and balances method available to ensure that work published in the academic forum is reasonable, well referenced, and well considered.

When you see peer-reviewed literature discussed on patient-generated websites or listserves, ask yourself if the persons assessing these articles are experts in the field or are individuals basing their opinions on their own experiences. In other words, who are these people? Does health blogger X or mom with disease Y have the academic credentials, training, or critical thinking skills needed to really assess scientific or medical peer-reviewed literature? Is it reasonable to think that blogger X or mom with disease Y has accurately interpreted the article? Only you can decide.

What Is Misinformation?

Misinformation means that some real facts are mixed with false statements, bias, or misapplied contexts or concepts. It can also mean that one fact is wrongly linked to another fact to create a completely false statement. Here are two examples:

- **Example 1.** Laboratory research in cell culture is misread as a legitimate therapy in humans. Lots of interesting laboratory results are years away from practical bedside application. Bench, or laboratory, research is not the same as bedside, or clinical, research. Many articles are misconstrued in this manner. People may read that some chemical component of a particular food delayed the growth of cancer cells in cell culture, then leap to the conclusion that this food will prevent cancer in everyone who eats it.
- **Example 2.** In the thyroid world, pharmaceutical companies are the source of funding for many kinds of research and educational conferences. These are called unrestricted educational grants, which are fully disclosed on conference materials. The grants go to the professional associations to pay for the tremendous costs of putting on an annual conference that reports on the latest research in that field. These educational conferences help physicians accrue Continuing Medical Education credits, keep up to date, and keep their licenses renewed. Researchers and clinicians who present at professional thyroid conferences such as the American Thyroid Association (ATA) annual meeting are not directly funded by the pharmaceutical companies supporting the ATA conferences and are usually not paid speakers. But on one prominent thyroid website, all the conference presenters and speakers were posted online and said to be "in the pockets" of pharmaceutical companies for simply presenting their research to their peers at a medical conference. This confused a lot of thyroid patients into thinking that their personal doctors were being

paid a check by a pharaceutical company, and the only reason they were being prescribed "synthetic" thyroid hormone (see Chapter 10) was because the doctor was paid to do so. This is the danger of misinformation. When presenters are specifically paid by a pharmaceutical company to present a speech, that is a different story. In these cases, the speaker has an ethical obligation to disclose all sources of direct funding, and it is up to the public to decide if the speaker is unduly influenced.

There are many forms of misinformation, but the important thing to remember is that it mixes some truth with fiction.

Appendix B

Legitimate Thyroid Resources for Patients

Finding a Thyroid Specialist
General sites
American Association of Clinical Endocrinologists
aace.com

American Thyroid Association
thyroid.org

The Endocrine Society
hormone.org

Head and neck surgeons (for thyroid surgery)
American Academy of Otolaryngology—Head and Neck
Surgery
entnet.org

Eye specialists (for thyroid eye disease)
American Academy of Ophthalmopathy
aao.org

Thyroid Websites that are Accountable to the Public Trust
North America
American Association of Clinical Endocrinologists
aace.com

American Thyroid Association
thyroid.org

Thyroid Foundation of Canada
thyroid.ca

Global (Note: addresses are provided only in the absence of
an e-mail address or website)
European Thyroid Association
eurothyroid.com

Latin American Thyroid Society
lats.org

*Patient Organizations (members of Thyroid Federation
International [TFI])*

Australia
Australian Thyroid Foundation
thyroidfoundation.com.au
Thyroid Australia
thyroid.org.au

Brazil
Thyroid Foundation of Brazil
E-mail: medneto@uol.com.br

Denmark
Thyreoidea Landsforeningen
thyreoidea.dk

Finland
Thyroid Foundation of Finland
www.kolumbus.fi/kilpirauhasliitto

France
l'Association Française des Malades de la Thyroïde
www.thyro-asso.org

Germany
Schilddrüsen Liga Deutschland e.V. (SLD)
schilddruesenliga.de

Italy
Associazione Italiana Basedowiani e Tiroidei
E-mail: emma99@libero.it

Japan
Thyroid Foundation of Japan
www.hata.ne.jp/tfj/

The Netherlands
Schildklierstichting Nederland
www.schildklier.nl

Norway

Norsk Thyreoideaforbund

www.stoffskifte.org

Republic of Georgia

Georgian Union of Diabetes and Endocrine Associations

E-mail: diabet@access.sanet.ge

Sweden

Sköldkörtelförening i Stockholm

skoldkortelforeningen.se

Västsvenska Patientföreningen för Sköldkörtelsjuka

vpfs.info

United Kingdom

British Thyroid Foundation

btf-thyroid.org

Graves' Disease

National Graves' Disease Foundation

ngdf.org

Parathyroid Gland

Parathyroid.com

parathyroid.com

This site is maintained by Dr. James Norman, a parathyroid surgeon.

Hypoparathyroidism

Hypoparathyroidism Association

hypoparathyroidism.org

This site is helpful if you have calcium problems after thyroid surgery.

Thyroid Eye Disease

The TED Association

http://www.thyroid-fed.org/members/TED.html

Thyroid Cancer

Thyroidcancerhelp (on Yahoo, under Groups)

This is a listserve maintained by my husband, Dr. Kenneth B. Ain, director, University of Kentucky Thyroid Oncology Program. I am listing this here because as of this writing, it is the only physician-monitored listserve on thyroid cancer.

ThyCa, Inc. (The Thyroid Cancer Survivors' Association)

thyca.org

Note: The listserves/support groups on ThyCa are not monitored by any medical advisor.

Canadian Thyroid Cancer Support Group Inc. (Thry'vors)

thryvors.org.

Note: There are no physicians routinely monitoring Thry'vors listserves.

Low-Iodine Diet Information

The Low Iodine Diet Cookbook by Norene Gilletz

This cookbook is published by my own publishing company, Your Health Press, and is available at Amazon.com and other online bookstores or through Trafford publishing (1-888-232-4444). I am listing it here because this particular version of the low-iodine diet has proven successful through verification and testing, and its kitchen-tested recipes were developed by a culinary expert. It is the only cookbook (rather than recipe exchange) on the low-iodine diet available as of this writing. Thyroid oncologist Dr. Kenneth Ain (my husband) was the medical advisor on this book, and wrote the Introduction.

Information on Other Conditions or Complementary Therapies

By using Appendix A as a guide, you can search the Internet widely for more information about many topics discussed in this book. For more information about complementary therapies, start with a visit to the NIH program, the National Center for Complementary and Alternative Therapies at http://nccam.nih.gov/.

Glossary

Terms in *italics* are also in the glossary.

acute suppurative thyroiditis A rare form of bacterial *thyroiditis*, in which pus and inflammation occur; treated with antibiotics.

Adam's apple The *thyroid* cartilage.

amiodarone A potent medicine used to treat heart rhythm disturbances, infamous for causing different types of thyroid problems.

anaplastic thyroid cancer A very rare but aggressive, hard-to-treat thyroid cancer with poor outcomes. It accounts for about 1.6 percent of all thyroid cancers.

angina Chest pain due to blockages of the blood supply to the heart muscle.

antithyroid medication Drugs that are used to treat *Graves' disease* in some people by preventing the thyroid from manufacturing *thyroid hormone*, occasionally leading to a remission of *Graves' disease*. *Propylthiouracil* (PTU) and *methimazole* (Tapazole) are commonly used antithyroid drugs.

"apathetic hyperthyroidism"   *Hyperthyroidism* without clear symptoms of *thyrotoxicosis*. It is usually diagnosed in individuals over sixty.

arrhythmia   Disturbance of the heart rhythm.

atherosclerotic cardiovascular disease (ASCVD)   Refers to fatty blockages of blood vessels anywhere in the body that can put you at risk for heart attack or stroke.

atrial fibrillation   A disordered, rapid, irregular heart rhythm.

autoimmune   Self-immune or self-attacking.

autoimmune disease   A disease where the body attacks its own tissue.

autoimmune thyroid disease   A thyroid disease involving *thyroid antibodies* that attack the *thyroid gland*, as in *Hashimoto's thyroiditis* or *Graves' disease*.

autonomous toxic nodules (ATNs)   Lumps that make *thyroid hormone* on their own and that do not respond to *TSH*. Autonomous toxic nodules can be single nodules or multinodular.

benign   Noncancerous.

beta-blocker   A type of drug that blocks adrenaline and slows the heart rate. It is used in people with *thyrotoxicosis*.

body mass index (BMI)   The best measurement of appropriate weight, calculated by dividing your weight (in kilograms) by your height (in meters) squared.

bradycardia   Slow heartbeat; associated with *hypothyroidism*.

catecholamines   Adrenaline and related hormones.

congenital hypothyroidism   *Hypothyroidism* that is present from birth. If congenital hypothyroidism is untreated, it can lead to *cretinism*.

congestive heart failure   Weakening of the pumping of the heart.

cretinism Stunted physical and mental development due to severe *hypothyroidism* in childhood. Most often caused by *iodine deficiency* and found in underdeveloped regions of the world.

CT scan A scan using computerized axial tomography.

cyst A fluid-filled lump; usually *benign*.

Cytomel The brand name of liothyronine sodium, also known as L-T3 by physicians. It is the pharmaceutical version of *triiodothyronine* (T3).

differentiated thyroid cancer cells Cancer cells that retain the functional features of normal thyroid *follicular cells*.

euthyroid Normal thyroid function.

exophthalmometer An instrument that measures the degree to which the eyes protrude from the skull. It is used in people with *exophthalmos*.

exophthalmos Bulging, watery eyes. This is a symptom of *thyroid eye disease*.

fine needle aspiration (FNA) biopsy A procedure in which a very thin needle (27 gauge) attached to a plastic syringe is pushed through the skin and into a *nodule* while the syringe plunger is gently pulled back, taking out material from the nodule. This material is smeared on glass slides to be viewed under a microscope and evaluated by a pathologist.

FNA Fine needle aspiration.

follicular cells The cells that produce *thyroid hormone*; follicular cells have receptors for special hormones that control the *thyroid gland*.

follicular thyroid cancer A type of thyroid cancer that is usually treatable with surgery and *radioactive iodine* with very good outcomes. It accounts for about 10 percent of all thyroid cancers.

free T4   The only portion of all the *T4* that is able to be taken up into each body cell and do the job of effective *thyroid hormone.*

free T4 test   The appropriate blood test to measure *free T4* levels.

generalized anxiety disorder (GAD)   A psychiatric/psychological disorder in which one suffers from persistent worry and anxiety without any relief, despite good reasons for relief from such worry.

gestational hyperthyroidism   When *hyperthyroidism* develops during pregnancy.

gestational hypothyroidism   When *hypothyroidism* develops during pregnancy.

gestational thyroid disease   When a thyroid disease develops during pregnancy.

glycemic index (GI)   Measures the rate at which various foods convert to glucose, which is assigned a value of 100. Higher numbers indicate a more rapid absorption of glucose, which helps to distinguish simple carbohydrates (or simple sugars) from more complex, or nutrient-dense, carbohydrates (such as grains).

goiter   An enlarged *thyroid gland.*

goitrogens   Substances that can block *thyroid hormone* formation. These are found in a variety of foods, including cabbage or other foods from the Brassica family.

Graves' disease   An *autoimmune thyroid disease* that causes *hyperthyroidism.*

Graves' ophthalmopathy (GO)   Another term for *thyroid eye disease.*

Hashimoto's disease   Another term for *Hashimoto's thyroiditis.*

Hashimoto's thyroiditis   A major cause of *hypothyroidism*, this type of *thyroiditis* is an *autoimmune thyroid disease* in which antibodies attack the *thyroid gland*, causing it to become inflamed, leak out its *thyroid hormone*, and then shrivel up.

Hashitoxicosis   Common in the early part of *Hashimoto's disease*, this condition causes *thyroid hormone* to leak out from the gland, causing *thyrotoxicosis*.

high-density lipoprotein (HDL)   The "good" cholesterol. It should be at least 40 mg/dL.

hypercholesterolemia   High cholesterol.

hypertension   High blood pressure.

hyperthyroid   Overactive *thyroid gland*, usually causing *thyrotoxicosis*.

hypocalcemia   Low calcium levels, which can lead to debilitating symptoms.

hypoparathyroidism   When the *parathyroid glands* do not make sufficient amounts of *parathyroid hormone*, usually due to damage during thyroid surgery, resulting in *hypocalcemia*, which can be temporary or permanent.

hypothalamus   A part of the brain that is just above the *pituitary gland*, which helps control the *pituitary gland* and the *thyroid gland* by releasing thyrotropin releasing hormone (TRH*)*.

hypothyroid   Low or nonfunctioning *thyroid gland*, causing a range of debilitating symptoms associated with low energy and a slowing down of body cells.

I-123   One type of *iodine isotope* used in *thyroid scans*.

I-131   One type of *iodine isotope* used in *thyroid scans* and treatment.

iodine   A crucial element the *thyroid gland* needs to make *thyroid hormone*.

iodine deficiency   When not enough *iodine* from food is available to the *thyroid gland*; causes *hypothyroidism*, *goiter*, and, in children or infants, mental retardation, short stature, or *cretinism*.

isotope   An element, such as *iodine*, that is radioactive or unstable.

isthmus   The middle part of the *thyroid gland*.

levothyroxine sodium   *Thyroid hormone* replacement made by a pharmaceutical company in pill form. It is also known as L-T4 by physicians and *T4* by the public.

lobectomy   Surgical removal of one lobe of the *thyroid gland*.

low-density lipoprotein (LDL)   The "bad" cholesterol. It should be less than 100 mg/dL.

low-iodine diet   A special diet low in *iodine* (not sodium) that can maximize the sensitivity and accuracy of *radioactive iodine* scans or treatments for thyroid cancer.

lymph nodes   Small *nodules* containing small white blood cells that stimulate the immune system to fight infection. Cancer cells may grow in lymph nodes, which are removed during the course of thyroid cancer surgery.

malignant   Cancerous.

medullary thyroid cancer (MTC)   A type of thyroid cancer that can be genetically inherited; treated with surgery if caught early and usually followed up with genetic testing.

methimazole (Tapazole)   An *antithyroid medication* used to treat *hyperthyroidism*.

mild hypothyroidism   Another term for *subclinical hypothyroidism*.

millicurie   A unit of measurement used for dosing *radioactive iodine* for scans or treatment.

MRI   A scan using magnetic resonance imaging.

neck dissection   Performed during a *thyroidectomy*, where the surgeon removes any obvious tumor that has spread to *lymph nodes* in the neck.

nodules   Lumps.

obesity   A *body mass index* between 30 and 34.9.

orbital decompression surgery   A surgical procedure that removes bone from the eye socket and expands the area alongside the eyeball so that swollen tissue can move into it; a corrective surgery in cases of severe *thyroid eye disease.*

osteoporosis   Bone loss.

palpitations   Rapid, forceful heartbeat.

panic attack   A cascade of physical symptoms associated with adrenaline and the "flight or fight" response (feelings of nausea and vertigo, cold sweat, choking sensations, *palpitations*, and shakiness). Commonly caused by *thyrotoxicosis.*

papillary thyroid cancer   A type of thyroid cancer that is usually treatable with surgery and *radioactive iodine*, with very good outcomes. It accounts for about 80 percent of all thyroid cancers.

parathyroid gland   These glands are close to the *thyroid gland* and they make *parathyroid hormone* (PTH).

parathyroid hormone (PTH)   Hormone that causes the kidneys to retain calcium in the blood while releasing phosphorus into the urine. It also increases the activation of vitamin D, which enhances the absorption of calcium and phosphorus from food and beverages.

pituitary gland   Located in the brain. It acts as a thermostat for the body and makes *thyroid-stimulating hormone.*

postpartum thyroiditis   A general label referring to *silent thyroiditis* occurring after delivery, causing mild *hyperthyroidism* and a short-lived version of *Hashimoto's disease.*

propranolol   A commonly used *beta-blocker.*

proptosis   Protusion, or bulging, of the eyeball, associated with *thyroid eye disease.*

propylthiouracil (PTU)   An *antithyroid medication* used to treat *hyperthyroidism.*

radioactive iodine (RAI)   *Iodine* that is radioactive; also called an *isotope.*

RAI   *Radioactive iodine.*

Riedel's thyroiditis   The rarest form of *thyroiditis,* in which the *thyroid gland* is invaded by scar tissue, infiltrating throughout the gland and binding it to surrounding portions of the neck. It is usually treated with surgery.

salivary stones   The swelling of one or more salivary glands (located under the ears and under the lower jaw) due to partial blockage of the salivary ducts by dried saliva. These are a complication of *radioactive iodine* treatment for thyroid cancer.

silent thyroiditis   A form of *thyroiditis* so named because it avoids detection until symptoms of *thyrotoxicosis* (and sometimes *hypothyroidism* thereafter) become severe. It usually resolves on its own.

sleep deprivation   Being deprived of the recommended hours of sleep for healthy adults.

sleep disorder   A physical disorder that interrupts deep, restful sleep. Often not recognized by the sufferer, who may have *sleep deprivation.*

stable iodine   Normal, or nonradioactive, *iodine.*

subacute viral thyroiditis   Also called de Quervain's *thyroiditis,* this type of short-lived *thyroiditis* may be viral in origin. Symptoms are pain and inflammation of the thyroid and *thyrotoxicosis* for about six weeks.

subclinical hyperthyroidism   Mild *hyperthyroidism* with few or no symptoms of *thyrotoxicosis.*

subclinical hypothyroidism   *Hypothyroidism* that has not progressed very far, meaning that there are few or no symptoms.

T3   Short for *triiodothyronine.*

T4   Short for *thyroxine.*

tachycardia   Fast heartbeat (or racing heart). It is associated with *hyperthyroidism*.

technetium   A type of *isotope* used for *thyroid scans*.

Thyrogen   A pharmaceutically prepared version of *thyroid-stimulating hormone* made from recombinant DNA technology. It is used in *thyroid scans* and other tests for thyroid cancer patients.

thyroglobulin (Tg)   A protein that is unique to thyroid cells and is the early form of *thyroid hormone*.

thyroglobulin test (Tg test)   A test that measures the amount of *thyroglobulin* in the blood. It is a useful marker for thyroid cancer cells.

thyroid antibodies   White blood cells that target the *thyroid gland*, causing an *autoimmune disease*.

thyroid antibody testing   A blood test that checks for the presence of *thyroid antibodies*.

thyroidectomy   Surgical removal of the *thyroid gland*. The procedure can be total or partial.

thyroid extract   A preparation of dried, cleaned, powdered *thyroid gland*s from cows or pigs. This is also known as natural *thyroid hormone*.

thyroid eye disease (TED)   An eye disease causing bulging, grittiness, redness, double vision, and a range of other eye symptoms. It is also called *Graves' ophthalmopathy* (GO) or Graves' orbitopathy, and it tends to strike people with *Graves' disease*.

thyroid gland   A butterfly-shaped gland typically located in front of the windpipe (trachea) just above the midline bony notch in the top of the breastbone (sternal notch).

thyroid hormone   A hormone made by the *thyroid gland* that serves as the speed control for all body cells. Types of *thyroid hormone* are *thyroxine (T4)* and *triiodothyronine (T3)*.

thyroid hormone resistance (Refetoff Syndrome)   A rare, inherited disease that results in a person being born with a resistance to his or her own *thyroid hormone*. It is caused by a mutation in the gene that makes the receptor for *thyroid hormone*.

thyroid hormone suppression therapy   A high dosage of *levothyroxine sodium* for the purposes of suppressing *thyroid-stimulating hormone*.

thyroiditis   Inflammation of the *thyroid gland*. It usually causes *hypothyroidism*.

thyroid lobe   One side, or lobe, of the *thyroid gland*. As the gland is butterfly-shaped, a lobe would be one "wing."

thyroid scan   A test where an image or picture is taken using special cameras and substances that light up for the camera.

thyroid self-exam   A self-exam of the neck area, which can help find suspicious thyroid lumps or an enlargement of the *thyroid gland* that should be evaluated by a doctor.

thyroid-stimulating hormone (TSH)   A special hormone that controls the level of *thyroid hormone*. High or low *TSH* levels indicate thyroid function problems.

thyroid-stimulating immunoglobulin (TSI or TSA)   A *thyroid antibody* that sticks to the *thyroid-stimulating hormone* receptor instead of to TSH. Overstimulating the *thyroid gland* causes *Graves' disease* or, when sticking to parts of the eye muscle, causes *thyroid eye disease.*

thyroid storm   When symptoms of severe *thyrotoxicosis* can manifest into a storm of severe cardiovascular symptoms that warrant emergency attention and admission to an intensive care unit.

thyrotoxic   Describes someone who suffers from *thyrotoxicosis.*

thyrotoxic goiter   *Goiter*s associated with prolonged *thyrotoxicosis* caused by *Graves' disease* or *autonomous toxic nodules.*

thyrotoxicosis Too much *thyroid hormone* caused by *hyperthyroidism*. Overdose of *thyroid hormone replacement, autonomous toxic nodules,* and other types of thyroid conditions lead to a range of debilitating symptoms associated with overstressed, exhausted body cells causing a speeding up of bodily processes.

Thyrotropin-releasing hormone (TRH) A hormone made by the *hypothalamus* when *thyroid hormone* levels are low.

thyroxine (T4) The inactive form of *thyroid hormone*. It is called T4 because it contains four iodine atoms for each hormone molecule.

total T3 test The appropriate blood test to measure the amount of active *thyroid hormone*, or *T3*, levels.

toxic multinodular goiter When the *thyroid gland* forms multiple *nodules* that produce too much *thyroid hormone*.

triiodothyronine (T3) Made by the body's cells out of *T4*, this is the active *thyroid hormone* that activates genes and "does the job" of *thyroid hormone*.

TSH *Thyroid-stimulating hormone.*

TSH test A sensitive blood test that assesses whether *thyroid-stimulating hormone* levels are high or low by looking at the body's own natural "thermostat" for *thyroid hormone*.

ultrasound A device that uses high-frequency sound waves to produce an "echo picture" of structures in the body.

undifferentiated thyroid cancer cells Cancer cells that do not retain the functional features of normal thyroid *follicular cells*.

unipolar depression The most common type of depression, characterized by one low, flat mood. It is frequently a complication of *hypothyrodism*.

WBS Whole body scan.

whole body scan (WBS) A scan involving pictures of the whole body that are used to track thyroid cancer recurrence.

Bibliography

About.com. "Guide Compensation." Accessed July 30, 2008, from http://beaguide.about.com/compensation.htm.

Ain, K. B. "Management of Thyroid Cancer." In *Diseases of the Thyroid,* Braverman, L. E. ed., 287–317. Totowa, N.J.: Humana Press, Inc., 1997.

———. "Management of Undifferentiated Thyroid Cancer." *Best Practice & Research Clinical Endocrinology & Metabolism* 14, no. 4 (2000): 615–29.

———. "Thyroid Malignancies." In *Oncologic Therapies,* Vokes, E. E., and H. M. Golomb, eds., 977–1000. Berlin: Springer-Verlag, 1999.

———. "Unusual Types of Thyroid Cancer." *Reviews in Endocrine & Metabolic Disorders* 1, no. 3 (2000): 225–31.

———. "What Is the Low Iodine Diet and Why Do You Need It?" In *The Low Iodine Diet Cookbook*, Gilletz, N., 5–19. Toronto: Your Health Press, 2005.

Ain, K. B., et al. "Thyroid Hormone Levels Affected by Time of Blood Sampling in Thyroxine-Treated Patients." *Thyroid* 3, no. 2 (1993): 81–5.

Ain, K. B., and M. S. Rosenthal. *The Complete Thyroid Book.* New York: McGraw-Hill, 2005.

Appelhof, B. C., et al. "Combined Therapy with Levothyroxine and Liothyronine in Two Ratios, Compared with Levothyroxine Monotherapy in Primary Hypothyroidism: A Double-Blind, Randomized, Controlled Clinical Trial." *Journal of Clinical Endocrinology & Metabolism* 90 (2005): 2666–74.

Bartalena, L., and J. Robbins. "Thyroid Hormone Transport Proteins." *Clinics in Laboratory Medicine* 13, no. 3 (1993): 583–98.

Benua, R. S., and R. D. Leeper. "A Method and Rationale for Treating Metastatic Thyroid Carcinoma with the Largest Safe Dose of 131I." In: Medeiros-Neto G., and E. Gaitan, eds. *Frontiers in Thyroidology* 2 (1986): 1317–21.

Bunevicius, R., et al. "Effects of Thyroxine as Compared with Thyroxine plus Triiodothyronine in Patients with Hypothyroidism." *New England Journal of Medicine* 340, no. 6 (February 11, 1999).

———. "Thyroxine vs Thyroxine plus Triiodothyronine in Treatment of Hypothyroidism after Thyroidectomy for Graves' Disease." *Endocrine* 18 (2002): 129–33.

Clyde, P. W., et al. "Combined Levothyroxine plus Liothyronine Compared with Levothyroxine Alone in Primary Hypothyroidism: A Randomized Controlled Trial." *Journal of the American Medical Association* 290 (2003): 2952–58.

Cooper, D. S. "Antithyroid Drugs in the Management of Patients with Graves' Disease: An Evidence-Based Approach to Therapeutic Controversies." *Journal of Clinical Endocrinology & Metabolism* 88, no. 8 (2003): 3474–81.

Demers, L. M., and C. A. Spencer. "Laboratory Medicine Practice Guidelines: Laboratory Support for the Diagnosis and Monitoring of Thyroid Disease." *Clinical Endocrinology* 58, no. 2 (2003): 138–40.

Dong, B. J., et al. "Bioequivalence of Generic and Brand-Name Levothyroxine Products in the Treatment of Hypothyroidism." *Journal of the American Medical Association* 277, no. 15 (April 16, 1997): 1199–200.

Edwards, C. M., et al. "Psychological Well-Being of Patients on l-Thyroxine." *Clinical Endocrinology* 59, no. 2 (2003): 264–65.

Escobar-Morreale, H. F., et al. "Thyroid Hormone Replacement Therapy in Primary Hypothyroidism: A Randomized Trial Comparing L-Thyroxine plus Liothyronine with L-Thyroxine Alone." *Annals of Internal Medicine* 142 (2005): 412–24.

———. "Treatment of Hypothyroidism with Combinations of Levothyroxine plus Liothyronine." *Journal of Clinical Endocrinology & Metabolism* 90 (2005): 4946–54.

Garton, M., et al. "Effect of L-Thyroxine Replacement on Bone Mineral Density and Metabolism in Premenopausal Women." *Clinical Thyroidology* 8, no. 1 (January–April 1995).

Geffner, D. L., and J. M. Hershman. "Beta-Adrenergic Blockade for the Treatment of Hyperthyroidism." *American Journal of Medicine* 93, no. 1 (1992): 61–68.

Gharib, H. "Changing Concepts in the Diagnosis and Management of Thyroid Nodules." *Endocrinology and Metabolism Clinics of North America* 26, no. 4 (1997): 777–800.

Grozinsky-Glasberg, S., et al. "Thyroxine-Triiodothyronine Combination Therapy versus Thyroxine Monotherapy for Clinical Hypothyroidism: Meta-Analysis of Randomized Controlled Trials." *Journal of Clinical Endocrinology & Metabolism* 91 (2006): 2592–99.

Gruters, A., et al. "Neonatal Thyroid Disorders." *Hormone Research* 59, no. 1 (2003): 24–29.

Hegedus, L., et al. "Management of Simple Nodular Goiter: Current Status and Future Perspectives." *Endocrine Reviews* 24, no. 1 (2003): 102–32.

Heyerdahl, S., and B. Oerbeck. "Congenital Hypothyroidism: Developmental Outcome in Relation to Levothyroxine Treatment Variables." *Thyroid* 13, no. 11 (2003): 1029–38.

Hu, F. B., and W. C. Willett. "Optimal Diets for Prevention of Coronary Heart Disease." *Journal of the American Medical Association* 288, no. 20 (November 27, 2002): 2569–78.

Kaplan, M., et al. "In Search of the Impossible Dream? Thyroid Hormone Replacement Therapy That Treats All Symptoms in Hypothyroid Patients." *Journal of Clinical Endocrinology and Metabolism* 88, no. 10 (2003): 4540–42.

Kelner, K., and L. Helmuth. "Obesity—What Is to Be Done?" *Science* 299, no. 5608 (2003): 845.

Knobel, M., and G. Medeiros-Neto. "An Outline of Inherited Disorders of the Thyroid Hormone Generating System." *Thyroid* 13, no. 8 (2003): 771–801.

Knudsen, N., et al. "Risk Factors for Goiter and Thyroid Nodules." *Thyroid* 12, no. 10 (2002): 879–88.

Kraiem, Z., and R. S. Newfield. "Graves' Disease in Childhood." *Journal of Pediatric Endocrinology & Metabolism* 14, no. 3 (2001): 229–43.

Langley, R. W., and H. B. Burch. "Perioperative Management of the Thyrotoxic Patient." *Endocrinology & Metabolism Clinics of North America* 32, no. 2 (2003): 519–34.

LiVolsi, V. A. *Surgical Pathology of the Thyroid.* Philadelphia: W. B. Saunders Co., 1990.

Macchia, P. E., et al. "Molecular Genetics of Congenital Hypothyroidism." *Current Opinion in Genetics & Development* 9, no. 3 (1999): 289–94.

Maxon, H. R., and H. S. Smith. "Radioiodine-131 in the Diagnosis and Treatment of Metastatic Well Differentiated Thyroid Cancer." *Endocrinology & Metabolism Clinics of North America* 19, no. 3 (1990): 685–718.

Mazer, N. A. "Interaction of Estrogen Therapy and Thyroid Hormone Replacement in Postmenopausal Women." *Thyroid* 14, no. 1 (2004): 27–34.

McDermott, M. T. "Thyroid Disease and Reproductive Health." *Thyroid* 14, no. 1 (2004): 1–3.

Olveira, G., et al. "Altered Bioavailability Due to Changes in the Formulation of a Commercial Preparation of Levothyroxine in Patients with Differentiated Thyroid Carcinoma." *Clinical Endocrinology* 46 (June 1997): 707–11.

Pinchera, A., and F. Santini. "Is Combined Therapy with Levothyroxine and Liothyronine Effective in Patients with Primary Hypothyroidism?" *Nature Clinical Practice: Endocrinology & Metabolism* 1 (2005): 18–19.

Quadbeck, B., et al. "Long-Term Follow-up of Thyroid Nodule Growth." *Experimental and Clinical Endocrinology & Diabetes* 110, no. 7 (2002): 348–54.

Redmond, G. "Thyroid Dysfunction and Women's Reproductive Health." *Thyroid* 14, no. 134 (2004): 5–16.

Robbins, J. "Treatment of Thyroid Cancer in Childhood." Proceedings of a workshop. [Bethesda, MD]: National Institutes of Health. In:

Wartofsky, L., and D. Van Nostrand, eds. *Thyroid Cancer.* New York: Springer-Verlag/Humana Press, 2006.

Rodriguez, T., et al. "Substitution of Liothyronine at a 1:5 Ratio for a Portion of Levothyroxine: Effect on Fatigue, Symptoms of Depression, and Working Memory versus Treatment with Levothyroxine Alone." *Endocrine Practice* 11 (2005): 223–33.

Rosenthal, M. S. *The Depression Sourcebook.* New York: McGraw-Hill, 2000.

———. "Ethical Problems with Patient Misconceptions in RAI Scans and Therapy." *Journal of Nuclear Medicine Technology* 34, no. 3 (2006): 143–50.

———. "The Impaired Hypothyroid Patient: Ethical Considerations and Obligations." *Thyroid* 17, no. 12 (2007): 1261–67.

———. *The Thyroid Cancer Book,* 2nd edition. Lexington, KY: Your Health Press, 2003.

———. *Women Managing Stress.* Toronto: Penguin Canada, 2002.

Rosenthal, M. S., and H. Pierce. "Inherited Medullary Thyroid Cancer and the Duty to Warn: Revisiting Pate v. Threlkel." *Thyroid* 15, no. 5 (2005): 140–45.

Rovet, J., and D. Daneman. "Congenital Hypothyroidism: A Review of Current Diagnostic and Treatment Practices in Relation to Neuropsychologic Outcome." *Pediatric Drugs* 5, no. 3 (2003): 141–49.

Sachiko, T., et al. "Dietary Protein and Weight Reduction. A Statement for Healthcare Professionals from the Nutrition Committee of the Council on Nutrition, Physical Activity, and Metabolism of the American Heart Association." *Circulation* 104 (2001): 1869–74.

Saravanan, P., et al. "Partial Substitution of Thyroxine (T4) with Tri-Iodothyronine in Patients on T4 Replacement Therapy: Results of a Large Community-Based Randomized Controlled Trial." *Journal of Clinical Endocrinology and Metabolism* 90 (2005): 805–12.

———. "Psychological Well-Being in Patients on 'Adequate' Doses of l-Thyroxine: Results of a Large, Controlled Community-Based Questionnaire Study." *Clinical Endocrinology* 57, no. 5 (November 2002): 577–78.

————. "Twenty-Four Hour Hormone Profiles of TSH, Free T3, and Free T4 in Hypothyroid Patients on Combined T3/T4 Therapy." *Experimental and Clinical Endocrinology & Diabetes* 115 (2007): 261–67.

Sawka, A. M., et al. "Does a Combination Regimen of T4 and T3 Improve Depressive Symptoms Better than T4 Alone in Patients with Hypothyroidism? Results of a Double-Blind, Randomized Controlled Trial." *Journal of Clinical Endocrinology and Metabolism* 88, no.10 (2003): 4551–55.

Siegmund, W., et al. "Replacement Therapy with Levothyroxine Plus Triiodothyronine (Bioavailable Molar Ratio 14:1) Is Not Superior to Thyroxine Alone to Improve Well-Being and Cognitive Performance in Hypothyroidism." *Clinical Endocrinology* 60, no. 6 (2004): 750–57.

Singer, P. A., et al. "Treatment Guidelines for Patients with Hyperthyroidism and Hypothyroidism." Standards of Care Committee, American Thyroid Association. *Journal of the American Medical Association* 273 (1995): 808–12.

Toft, A. "Thyroid Hormone Replacement—One Hormone or Two?" *New England Journal of Medicine* 340, no. 6 (February 11, 1999).

Walsh, J., et al. "Combined Thyroxine/Liothyronine Treatment Does Not Improve Well-Being, Quality of Life, or Cognitive Function Compared to Thyroxine Alone: A Randomized Controlled Trial in Patients with Primary Hypothyroidism." *Journal of Clinical Endocrinology and Metabolism* 88, no. 10 (2003): 4543–50.

Weiss, R. E., and S. Refetoff. "Resistance to Thyroid Hormone." *Reviews in Endocrine and Metabolic Disorders* 1, no. 1–2 (2000): 97–108.

Whitley, R. J., and K. B. Ain. "Thyroglobulin: A Specific Serum Marker for the Management of Thyroid Carcinoma." *Clinics in Laboratory Medicine* 24, no. 1 (2004): 29–47.

Williams, D. "Cancer After Nuclear Fallout: Lessons from the Chernobyl Accident." *Nature Reviews: Cancer* 2, no. 7 (2002): 543–49.

Index

About.com, 206
Academic journal articles, 203–4, 208
Acid reflux, 15
Acropachy, 37
Acupuncture, 93, 199, 200
Acute suppurative thyroiditis, 10, 61–62
Adam's apple, 65
Addison's disease, 120
Adenocarcinoma, 74–75
Adenomas, 64, 72, 76
Adrenaline, 34, 38, 54, 55, 105, 111
Adrenergic system, 34, 39
Aerobic activities, 187–88
Africa, 170, 171
Agar-agar, 174
Age
    fertility and, 122
    follicular thyroid cancer and, 86, 88
    Hashimoto's thyroiditis and, 25, 118
    Hurthle cell cancer and, 86
    hypothyroidism and, 10, 13, 21, 26,
        116, 118–19, 120
    papillary thyroid cancer and, 87–88
    sleep problems and, 114, 115
    thyroid disease after sixty, 118–20
Alcohol, 183
Algin, 174
Alginates, 174
Alopecia, 55, 56. *See also* Hair loss and
    changes
Alps, 170
Alternative therapies, xvi–xvii, 201

American Association of Clinical
    Endocrinologists (AACE), 21
American Society for Reproductive
    Medicine (ASRM), 122
American Thyroid Association (ATA), 22,
    30, 209
Amiodarone, 111, 164
Anaplastic thyroid cancer, 75, 87
Andes Mountains, 170
Anemia, 17, 120
    aplastic, 48
    pernicious, 13
Angina, 14, 106, 111–12, 119
Animal thyroid hormone, dried, 4–5, 10,
    154–57
Antacids, 163
Antidepressants, 133
Antithyroglobulin (TG) antibodies, 25
Antithyroid medication, 72
    breastfeeding and, 131
    for Graves' disease, 45, 46–49, 50,
        126, 127
    heart complications and, 111
    pregnancy and, 126, 127, 128, 129,
        136
Anxiety, 35, 36, 102–3, 105–6
Aplastic anemia, 48
Armour, 156, 157
Arrhythmias, 107, 111
Arthritis, 18, 40, 118. *See also*
    Rheumatoid arthritis
Asia, 171

Aspirin, 36, 59
Asthma, 55
Atenolol, 55
Atherosclerotic cardiovascular disease
    (ASCVD), 106–7, 110
Atkins diet, 181–82
Atrial fibrillation, 34, 38, 111
Autoimmune disease collection package,
    97, 120
Autoimmune disorders, 13, 26, 36, 97,
    120, 121, 172
Autoimmune thyroid disease, xv, 1, 10,
    36, 98, 120, 121, 122, 131. *See
    also* Graves' disease; Hashimoto's
    thyroiditis
Autonomous toxic nodules (ATNs), 51–
    52, 63, 66, 72, 73, 78, 146
Autosomal dominant gene disorders,
    82–83

Bamboo shoots, 173
Barnes, Broda O., 30–31
Basal body temperature test, 22, 30
Basal metabolic rate, 22
Bean sprouts, 173
Beans, 173
Belarus, Russia (radioactive fallout in), 82
Beta-adrenergic receptors, 55, 105
Beta-blockers, 34, 39, 41, 42, 54, 72, 89,
    111, 112
    anxiety/panic and, 105, 106
    breastfeeding and, 132
    cancer therapy and, 89
    de Quervain's thyroiditis and, 59
    Graves' disease and, 49, 50, 51
    during pregnancy, 128, 129–30
    side effects of, 55, 56
    silent thyroiditis and, 60
    thyroid eye disease (TED) and, 98, 100
Bikini Atoll, 82
Bile, 110
Bioidentical hormones, 117, 155
Biopsies. *See* Fine needle aspiration (FNA)
    biopsies
Bipolar disorder, 35, 36, 164
Birth defects, 151
Bladder infections, 182
Bladder wrack, 172
Blindness, 101
Blogs, xvi
Blood pressure, elevated. *See*
    Hypertension
Blood sugar, 39, 178–79, 181

Body Mass Index (BMI), 185
Bone fractures, osteoporosis-related, 116
Bowel movements, 35, 36, 183
Bradycardia, 108
Brassica vegetable family, 173
Brazil, 170
Bread, 175
Breast cancer, 81, 117, 151, 152
Breastfeeding, 129, 131, 132, 144
Brody, Jane E., xv
Bruising, 36
Burnout, 115–16
Bush, Barbara, 43
Bush, George H. W., 43
Butter, 175

C cells, 7–8, 86–87
Cabbage, 173
Caffeine, 183
Calcitonin, 7, 117
Calcitriol, 94
Calcium, 8, 93–94, 124, 162, 172, 183
Cancer. *See also* Thyroid cancer
    breast, 81, 117, 151, 152
    Hodgkin's disease, 23
    leukemia, 151–52
    lung, 81
    radioactive iodine-induced (myth),
        151–52
Carbohydrates, 179, 181–82, 184
Carcinoma, 64, 74
Cardiovascular/heart disease, 11, 14, 97,
    106–12, 193
    after sixty, 119
    atherosclerotic, 106–7, 110
    diet and, 182
    Graves' disease and, 43–44
    menopause and, 116
    obesity and, 108, 184
    similiarities to hypothyroidism, 119
    sleep apnea and, 115
Carotene, 19
Carpal tunnel syndrome, 18
Carrageenan, 174
Case studies
    anxiety or hyperthyroidism, 35
    dancing as weight loss method, 189
    depression, 107
    familial medullary thyroid cancer
        (FMTC), 84
    Graves' treatment, 145
    hair loss as beta-blocker side effect, 56
    Hashimoto's thyroiditis, 24

housework, getting help with, 196
Hurricane Katrina, 163
hypothyroidism or heart disease, 119
improper storage of medicine, 161
infertility, 123
low-iodine diet, 177
hypothyroid misdiagnosed as
    depression, 15
natural vs. synthetic hormones, 156
panic attacks or thyroid disorder, 42
pediatric cancer, 67
postpartum thyroiditis, 61
post-RAI treatment precautions, 147
posttreatment hypothyroidism, 47
pregnancy and Graves' disease, 127
RAI concerns, 149
smoking and thyroid eye disease (TED),
    99
talk therapy, 198
T4/T3 conversion myth, 4–5
unusual case of Graves' disease, 28
Cassava, 173
Catecholamines, 34, 111
Cauliflower, 173
Celiac disease, 27
Central sleep apnea, 114
Chatrooms, xvi
Chen, Amy, 152
Chernobyl reactor accident, 77, 82, 137
Chest pain, 14, 106, 111–12
Children. *See also* Infants and newborns
    acute suppurative thyroiditis in, 61–62
    Graves' disease in, 43
    medication monitoring for, 162
    obesity in, 185
    radiation therapy and, 64, 68
    radioactive fallout exposure, 77–78, 82
    thyroid cancer in, 67, 81, 82
China, 170
Chocolate, 175
Cholesterol levels, 163, 181, 183, 186
    exercise and, 188
    high-density lipoprotein, 188
    hypothyroidism and, 14, 17, 108, 110,
        118
    low-density lipoprotein, 110, 179–80,
        182, 188
Cholestyramine, 163
Chronic fatigue syndrome, 26
Clinical (bedside) research, 209
Coffee, 161
Cognitive behavioral therapy, 106
Cold intolerance, 14

Cold nodules, 68, 141
Cold phase of thyroid eye disease (TED),
    100
Colestipol, 163
Colloid nodules, 63, 66, 71
Combination therapy (T3/T4), 119, 155,
    157, 167–68
Complementary therapies, xix, 12, 187–
    201. *See also* Acupuncture; Exercise;
    Massage; Meditation; Mental health
Complications and comorbidities,
    11, 97–120. *See also* Anxiety;
    Cardiovascular/heart disease;
    Depression; Fatigue; Menopause;
    Sleep disorders; Thyroid eye disease
    (TED)
Computerized tomography (CT), 95, 101,
    102, 142
Concentration problems, 18
Congestive heart failure, 39, 106, 108–9,
    111, 119
Constipation, 15, 16, 36, 178, 179, 182,
    184, 187
Conversion of T4 to T3, 3, 4–6, 22, 112,
    153, 154, 165, 167, 172
Copper sulfur, 172
Corneal ulcers, 100
Cortisone, 59
Counseling/Counselors, 195–97. *See also*
    Talk therapy
Cramps, 18
C-reactive protein (CRP), 59
Cretinism, 170
Critical thinking skills, 205–9
Cured and corned foods, 175
Cysts, 63, 64, 66, 71–72
    cyst sclerosis, 72
Cytomel, 142, 153, 164

Dairy products, 124, 140, 174, 183
Dancing, 188, 189
De Quervain's (subacute viral) thyroiditis,
    10, 57–59, 60
Deafness, 135
Deep tissue massage, 199
Deiodinases, 3
Dementia, 118
Depression, 11, 36, 97, 102–5, 107, 115,
    164
    bipolar, 35, 36, 164
    hyperthyroidism and, 14–15, 35
    hypothyroidism and, 14–15, 26, 35,
        102–5, 118

managing, 105
postpartum (*see* Postpartum blues;
    Postpartum depression)
postprandial, 184
sadness vs., 104
situational, 103
symptoms of, 104–5
unipolar, 103–5
Diabetes, 110
    Graves' disease and, 44
    obesity and, 183, 184, 186
    Type 1 (insulin-dependent), 13, 26, 44,
        120, 127
    Type 2, 44, 120, 179, 183, 184, 186
Diet and nutrition, 169–86
    carbohydrates in, 179, 181–82, 184
    fats in, 110, 181–82
    fiber in, 178, 179–80
    iodine in (*see* Iodine, dietary)
    weight loss and, 181–83
Diet of poverty, 186
Digestive changes, 15–16
Dihydrotachysterol, 94
Dosimetry, 96, 148
Driving, contraindications to, 19, 142,
    150

Eclampsia, 128
Ectopic thyroid, 134–35
Edema, 37, 108, 199
Eggs, 6, 174
Emphysema, 55
Endocrinologists, xviii–xix
Endorphins, 187, 200
Energy drains, eliminating, 193–95
Epinephrine. *See* Adrenaline
Erythrocyte sedimentation rate (ESR), 59
Estrogen, 17–18, 40, 116, 117, 125, 155
Europe, 144, 151, 171
Euthyroid Graves' disease, 51
Euthyroidism, 17, 21
Exercise, 186, 187–91
Exhaustion, 37. *See also* Fatigue
Exophthalmometer, 101
Exophthalmos, 98
External beam radiation therapy (EBRT),
    23, 77, 78, 82
    author's treatment, xiv
    indications for, 89, 96
Eye disease. *See* Thyroid eye disease
    (TED)
Eyes, watering of the, 149

Familial hypercholesterolemia, 110
Familial medullary thyroid cancer
    (FMTC), 83, 84, 86
Family history. *See* Genetic factors
Fatigue, 10, 11, 16, 112–15, 187. *See also*
    Exhaustion
    misinformation about, 112
    normal, 113
Fats, dietary, 110, 181–82
Fertility and fertility problems, 11, 39, 40,
    54, 122–24
Fetal thyrotoxicosis, 126
Fiber, 178, 179–80
Fibromyalgia, 26
Fine needle aspiration (FNA) biopsies, 66,
    67, 68–70, 130, 141
    accuracy of, 69–70
    confirming a pathology report, 70
    of cysts, 71–72
    of multinodular goiters, 74
Fingernail changes, 16, 37
Fingertip changes, 37
Fish, 6, 174, 175, 177
5-prime deiodinase, 3, 22
Flavenoids, 173
Follicular cells, 7
Follicular neoplasia, 76
Follicular thyroid cancer, 11, 75, 85–86,
    95, 146
    anaplastic, 87
    iodine excess and, 172
    staging, 88
    treatment of, 89, 90
    treatment of recurrence, 96
Food. *See* Diet and nutrition
Food and Drug Administration (FDA),
    117, 143
Free T4 levels, 3, 112
Free T4 test, 20, 26, 44, 53, 95, 135
Free T3 test, 44, 53

Generalized anxiety disorder (GAD), 105
Generic drugs, 158–59
Genetic factors
    in cholesterol levels, 110
    in hypertension, 109
    in hypothyroidism, 13
    in obesity, 186
    in thyroid cancer, 82–83, 87
Genetic screening, 83, 87
Gestational hypertension, 128
Gestational hyperthyroidism, 11, 129–30

Gestational hypothyroidism. *See*
  Hypothyroidism, pregnancy and
Gestational thyroid disease, 126–30
Gestational thyrotoxicosis, 124, 128
Gestational trophoblastic neoplasia,
  128
Glycemic index, 178–79, 181
Goiter belts, 170
Goiters, 10–11, 16, 36–37
  de Quervain's thyroiditis and, 59
  Graves' disease and, 43, 44, 46, 48,
    49, 129
  Hashimoto's thyroiditis and, 23,
    25–26, 118
  iodine deficiency and, 6, 12, 170
  iodine excess and, 6, 171
  lithium and, 164
  multinodular (*see* Multinodular goiters)
  in newborns, 136
  Pendred syndrome and, 135
  sleep apnea and, 113, 114
  thyroiditis and, 57
Goitrogenic diets, 46
Goitrogens, 173
Graves, Robert James, 43
Graves' disease, 10, 16, 33, 35, 42, 43–51,
  58, 66, 78, 120, 131, 191
  after sixty, 120
  cause of, 43
  complications of, 43–44
  diagnosis of, 44–45
  euthyroid, 51
  Hashimoto's thyroiditis compared
    with, 24
  heart complications and, 111
  lithium and, 164
  natural course of, 51
  pregnancy and, 46, 121, 122, 126, 127,
    129, 130, 131, 136
  radioactive iodine therapy for, 45, 46,
    48–49, 50, 78, 137, 138, 139,
    144–45, 147, 150–51, 153
  relapse, 47
  remission of, 47–48, 49–50, 72
  smoking and, 98–99
  thyroid eye disease (TED) and, 11, 37,
    43, 44, 46, 48, 51, 97, 98–99
  treating thyrotoxicosis not caused by,
    54–55
  treatment of, 45–49, 145
  unusual case of, 28
Great Lakes region, 170

Greece, 170
Ground nuts, 173

Hair loss and changes, 15, 17, 37–38, 44,
  55, 56, 152
Hamburger toxicosis, 53
Hanford nuclear facility, 82
Hashimoto, Hakaru, 23
Hashimoto's thyroiditis, 9, 10, 16, 21,
  23–26, 43, 54, 57, 59–60, 120, 189,
  196
  age and, 25, 118
  cause of, 23
  de Quervain's thyroiditis compared
    with, 58–59
  diagnosis of, 25
  iodine excess and, 172
  postpartum, 131, 132
  pregnancy and, 121, 126, 127, 130
  thyroid eye disease (TED) and, 24, 97
  treatment of, 25–26
Hashitoxicosis, 24–25, 54, 58, 60
Health narrative, 207–8
Heart attacks, 106, 108, 109, 110, 112,
  115, 183
Heart disease. *See* Cardiovascular/heart
  disease
Heart failure, 14, 111. *See also* Congestive
  heart failure
Heart palpitations, 38–39, 111
Heart rate, 38. *See also* Pulse rate; Racing
  heart
Heartburn, 15
Heat intolerance, 38
Henrik, Per, 199
Herbal supplements, 172
High-density lipoprotein (HDL)
  cholesterol, 188
High-output congestive heart failure, 111
Himalayas, 170
Hiroshima (atomic bombing of), 77, 137
Hodgkin's disease, 23
Hormone replacement therapy (HRT) for
  menopause, 117, 155, 156
Hot nodules, 66, 68, 72, 74, 141
Hot phase of thyroid eye disease (TED),
  100
Human chorionic gonadotropin (HCG),
  128
Hurthle cell (oncocytic) cancer, 75, 86
Hydatidiform mole, 128
Hydroxypyridines, 173

Hyperdefecation, 36, 183
Hypertension
  gestational, 128
  hypothyroidism and, 14, 108, 109–10
  low-carb diets and, 182
  obesity and, 186
  sleep apnea and, 115
Hyperthyroidism, 1, 10, 14–15, 35,
    36–37, 73, 123, 139, 143, 153
  after sixty, 118, 120
  amiodarone-induced, 164
  defined, 33
  diagnosing, 53–54
  diet and, 173, 183
  gestational, 11, 129–30
  Graves' disease (*see* Graves' disease)
  in infants and newborns, 136
  ketosis and, 182
  lithium and, 164
  menopause and, 116
  postpartum, 131
  thyrotoxicosis distinguished from, 33
  thyrotoxicosis from causes other than,
    51–53
  weight loss and, 184
Hypocalcemia, 94
Hypoglycemia, 39
Hypoparathyroidism, 93–94
Hypoplastic thyroid gland, 135
Hypothalamus, 7, 27, 135
Hypothyroid withdrawal preparation, 19,
    142, 147, 165–66
Hypothyroidism, 1, 13–32, 35, 102–5,
    112, 113, 153, 191
  after sixty, 118–19, 120
  amiodarone-induced, 164
  burnout and, 115–16
  causes of, 21–27
  de Quervain's thyroiditis and, 59
  diagnosis of, 19–21
  diet and, 173, 178–80, 182
  exercise and, 187
  heart disease and, 14, 106, 108–10
  hidden, 28–31
  iatrogenic, 13, 21–23
  in infants and newborns, 21, 134–36,
    170, 171
  iodine excess and, 172
  lithium-induced, 164
  massage and, 198, 199
  menopause and, 116
  obesity and, 184–85
  overview, 9–10

  postpartum, 131
  posttreatment, 47
  pregnancy and, 11, 26, 122, 124, 125,
    127–28
  primary, 13, 21–23
  risk factors for, 13
  silent thyroiditis and, 60
  subclinical (*see* Subclinical
    hypothyroidism)
  symptoms of, 14–19
  symptoms with normal tests, 27–32
  T3 for severe, 166–67
  as a therapeutic goal, 45, 46, 47, 50,
    93, 144–45, 150–51
  thyroid eye disease (TED) and, 100
  thyroiditis and, 57
  treatment of, 27, 118–19
  untreated Graves' disease and, 51
  yoga and, 190

I-123, 138, 140
I-131, 138, 140, 143–45, 146, 147, 148
Iatrogenic hypothyroidism, 13, 21–23
Immune system, 130–31, 172
Impotence, 40
Infants and newborns, 121, 133–36
  athyreotic, 21, 135
  hyperthyroidism in, 136
  hypothyroidism in, 21, 134–36, 170,
    171
  iodine deficiency in, 170, 171
Infertility. *See* Fertility and fertility
    problems
Informed consent, 46, 145
Insoluble fiber, 179, 180
Insomnia, 115
Insulin, 44, 179, 182
Insulin resistance, 181
International Council for Control
    of Iodine Deficiency Disorders
    (ICCIDD), 171
Internet, xv–xvii, xviii
  on conversion of T4 to T3, 4–5
  credible information sources on, 205
  health narrative on, 207–8
  medical literature search guidelines,
    204
  support groups on, 192
  on thyroid hormone resistance, 29–30
Iodate dough conditioners, 175
Iodine
  in amiodarone, 111, 164
  conversion of T4 to T3, 3

deficiency of, 6, 12, 21, 134, 170–71
dietary, 6, 140, 169–78 (*see also* Low-
    iodine diet)
excess of, 136, 171, 172
pregnancy and, 124, 127, 171
thyroid failure to take up, 135
TSH and, 7, 171
Iron, 125, 162, 172
Isthmus, 2, 91

Japan, 144, 151

Kelp, 140, 171, 172, 174
Kennedy, John F., 43
Ketosis, 182
Kidneys, 8, 93, 94, 109–10, 142, 143, 182
Kohlrabi, 173

Laboratory (bench) research, 204, 209
Lactation, 124. *See also* Breastfeeding
Lactose intolerance, 183
Latin America, 171
Leukemia, 151–52
Levothyroxine, 4, 15, 26, 50, 53, 76,
    110, 153, 154–55, 156, 157. *See also*
    Thyroid hormone replacement
dosing, 159–60
misconceptions/myths about, 30, 31
for newborns, 134
for nodule shrinking, 74
pre-scan discontinuation of, 142
Lid lag, 100
Lid retraction, 98
Light of Life Foundation, 176
Lima beans, 173
Listserves, xvi, 208
Lithium, 27, 164
Lobectomy, 72, 89, 90, 91
Lobectomy and isthmusectomy, 91
Lobes, thyroid, 2
London Medical and Surgical Journal, 43
Low-carbohydrate diets, 181–82
Low-density lipoprotein (LDL)
    cholesterol, 110, 179–80, 182, 188
Low-fat diets, 181
Low-iodine diet, 12, 90, 94, 141–42, 143,
    147, 169–70, 173–78
brief history of, 174
daily total intake on, 174, 176
duration of, 176–78
inaccurate/unproven versions, 175–76
restrictions on, 174–75
Low Iodine Diet Cookbook (Gilletz), 177

Lung cancer, 81
Lupus, 13, 26, 120
Lymph nodes, cancer spread to, 86, 89,
    148. *See also* Neck dissection
Lymphedema, 108
Lymphocytes, 23, 59
Lymphocytic thyroiditis, 59

Magnesium, 172
Magnetic resonance imaging (MRI), 95,
    101, 102
Maize, 173
Manganese, 172
Mania, 35
Manual lymph drainage, 199
Margarine, 175
Marriage and family counselors, 197
Marshall Islands, 77, 82, 137
Massage, 93, 198–200
Medical review of articles, 206, 207
Medication
improper storage of, 161
Meditation, 200–201
Medullary thyroid cancer (MTC), 8, 11,
    75
familial, 83, 84, 86–87
Memory problems, 18, 118
Men
de Quervain's thyroiditis in, 58
depression in, 104
Graves' disease in, 43
Hashimoto's thyroiditis in, 23
hypothyroidism in, 13
infertility and, 122
normal TSH levels in, 20
panic attacks in, 54
thyroid cancer in, 81, 85, 86
thyrotoxicosis in, 40
Menopause, 11, 25, 26, 38, 116–17, 155.
    See also Perimenopause
Menstrual cycle, 17, 40
Mental health, 191–97. *See also specific
    disorders*
Mental retardation, 12, 134, 170
Methimazole, 46, 129, 136, 173
Metoprolol, 55
Mexico, 170
MIBI scans, 95
Milk, 6, 78, 176, 183
Milky discharge from breasts, 17–18
Millet, 173
Miscarriage, 39, 54, 122, 123, 129, 130
Misinformation, 209–10. *See also* Myths

Molar pregnancy, 128
Molasses, 175
Morning sickness, 124–25, 128
Multinodular goiters, 11
    nontoxic, 73–74
    toxic, 51, 52, 63, 73–74, 138
Muscle aches, 18
Muscle weakness, 40
Myasthenia gravis, 40, 120
Myocardial infarction, 106. *See also*
    Heart attacks
Myths. *See also* Misinformation
    of the benign multinodular goiter,
        73–74
    on herbal supplements, 172
    on hypothyroidism, 29–32
    on radioactive iodine, 150–52
    on T4/T3 conversion, 4–5, 112
    on TSH suppression by T3, 22
Myxedema, 15, 19, 44, 154, 166

Nagasaki (atomic bombing of), 77, 137
National Cancer Institute, 77, 82
National Graves' Disease Foundation, 137
National Institutes of Health (NIH), 174,
    176
Neck dissection, xiv, 89, 90, 91
Nerve damage, 93
Netherlands, 170
Neuromuscular massage, 199
Nevada Test Site, 82
New York Times, xv
Nodulectomy, 76
Nodules, thyroid, 11, 45, 63–79, 139
    autonomous toxic, 51–52, 63, 66, 72,
        73, 78, 146
    benign, 71–72
    cold, 68, 141
    colloid, 63, 66, 71
    evaluating, 66
    finding, 64–65
    hot, 66, 68, 72, 74, 141
    indeterminate or suspicious, 75–76
    malignant, 74–75
    out-of-date approaches for shrinking,
        74
    pregnancy and, 121, 130
    screening criteria, 77–79
    sleep apnea and, 113, 114
    types of, 70–76
Nontoxic multinodular goiters, 73–74
Noradrenaline/norepinephrine, 34
Numbness, 18, 93

Oak Ridge atomic laboratory, 138
Obesity, 109, 179, 183–86. *See also*
    Weight gain
    biological causes of, 185–86
    heart disease and, 108, 184
    sleep apnea and, 115
Obstructive sleep apnea, 114–15
Olive oil, 175
Onycholysis, 37
Orbital decompression surgery,
    102
Osteoblasts, 117
Osteoclasts, 117
Osteoporosis, 8, 40, 116–17, 119
Ovulation, 17, 18, 39, 40

Pancreatitis, 182
Panic attacks/disorder, 35, 39, 42, 54,
    105–6
Papillary thyroid cancer, 11, 75, 85,
    91, 95, 146
    anaplastic, 87
    iodine excess and, 172
    staging, 87–88
    tall cell, xiv, 85, 89
    treatment of, 89–90
    treatment of recurrence, 96
Parafollicular cells, 7–8, 86–87
Parathyroid glands, 8–9, 93–94, 162
Parathyroid hormone (PTH), 8, 93
Peer-reviewed literature, 204, 206, 207,
    208–9
Pendred syndrome, 135
Pendrin protein, 135
Perimenopause, 26, 53–54, 116
Periorbital edema, 37
Peripheral vascular disease, 107, 184
Peripheral vascular resistance, 109
Pernicious anemia, 13
PET scans, 95
Pets, 193
Pharmaceutical companies, 206, 209–10
Phosphorus, 8
Pig thyroid hormone. *See* Animal thyroid
    hormone, dried
Pituitary gland, 3, 20, 23, 25, 43, 63, 72,
    73, 166
    disorders and diseases of, 27
    iodine deficiency and, 170
    in newborns, 135
    role of TSH and, 6–7
    tumors of, 4
Plutonium, 82

Poland (radioactive fallout in), 77–78, 82
Postpartum blues, 131, 132–33
Postpartum depression, 26, 60, 131, 133
Postpartum thyroiditis, 10, 60–61, 122, 127, 131–33
Postprandial depression, 184
Potassium iodide tablets, 78, 82
Prednisone, 59, 102
Preeclampsia, 128
Pregnancy, 11–12, 26, 110, 120, 123–30, 184. *See also* Fertility and fertility problems
   Graves' disease and, 46, 121, 122, 126, 127, 129, 130, 136
   iodine during, 124, 127, 171
   low-carb diets and, 182
   molar, 128
   normal discomforts of, 124–25
   preexisting thyroid disease and, 121, 125–26
   radioactive iodine scans and, 142
   radioactive iodine therapy and, 123–24, 144, 151
Premature delivery, 122, 128
Premenstrual syndrome (PMS), 26, 53–54
Pretibial myxedema, 44
Progesterone, 117
Prolactin, 17–18
Propranolol, 55, 128, 129–30, 136
Proptosis, 37, 98
Propylthiouracil (PTU), 46, 48, 128, 129, 136
Psychiatric misdiagnosis, 14–15, 34–36
Psychologists/psychological associates, 195, 197
PTU. *See* Propylthiouracil (PTU)
PubMed, 203, 204
Pulse rate, 14, 35, 39, 111, 119

Qi, 190, 200
Qigong, 190–91

Racing heart, 43, 111
Radiation exposure, 77–79, 83, 85–86
Radioactive fallout, 68, 77–78, 81–82, 137
Radioactive iodine (RAI), 137–52
   discovery of, 138
   nuclear testing with, 139–43
   properties and uses of, 138–39

Radioactive iodine (RAI) scans, 12, 138–39, 140–43
   for autonomous toxic nodules (ATNs), 52, 72, 78, 146
   breastfeeding and, 131
   for de Quervain's thyroiditis, 59
   for differentiated vs. undifferentiated cancer, 88
   for Graves' disease, 45, 78
   hot and cold areas on, 140
   low risks associated with, 78
   for nodules, 66, 139, 141
   preparation for, 165–66
   for silent thyroiditis, 60
   for thyroid cancer, 94, 140, 141–43, 165–66, 170
   for toxic multinodular goiters, 52, 73–74
   unnecessary, 139, 141
   whole body, 138, 141–43, 148, 165
Radioactive iodine (RAI) therapy, 12, 22, 143–52
   author's treatment, xiv
   for autonomous toxic nodules (ATNs), 72, 73
   breastfeeding and, 131
   in childhood, 64, 68
   for follicular thyroid cancer, 86, 146
   for Graves' disease, 45, 46, 48–49, 50, 78, 137, 138, 139, 144–45, 147, 150–51, 153
   for hyperthyroidism, 143
   low risks associated with, 78
   misconceptions about, 150–52
   for papillary thyroid cancer, 90, 146
   posttreatment precautions, 146, 147, 149–50
   pregnancy and, 123–24, 144, 151
   preparing for, 146–47, 165–66
   side effects of, 148
   standard dosing, 147–48
   for thyroid cancer, 86, 89, 90, 92, 94–95, 138, 139, 143, 146–50, 165–66, 170
   thyroid eye disease (TED) and, 102
   for toxic multinodular goiters, 74
Radioactive iodine (RAI) uptake tests, 139–40
Radioactive isotopes, 138, 140
Radioactive thallium scans, 95
Rapid eye movement (REM) sleep, 114
Red food dye (FD&C Red Dye #3), 174, 175

Refetoff Syndrome, 29. *See also* Thyroid hormone resistance
Remission of Graves' disease, 47–48, 49–50, 72
Restless legs syndrome (RLS), 115
Review articles, 204, 205
Rheumatoid arthritis, 13, 26, 120
Riedel's thyroiditis, 10, 62

Saliva decrease, 148
Salivary stones, 148–49
Salt, 140, 171, 174, 175
Sargassum, 172
Seafood, 140, 174
Selenium, 172
Sexual function and libido, 40–41
Shellfish, 6
Shiatsu massage, 199
Silent thyroiditis, 10, 59–60, 131, 132
Situational depression, 103
Size
    of autonomous toxic nodules (ATNs), 73
    of cysts, 71–72
    of nodules, 64
    of thyroid cancer, 75, 89
Skin changes, 18–19, 41
Sleep, 16, 112–15
Sleep apnea, 84, 113, 114–15, 118
Sleep deprivation, 113–14
Sleep disorders, 11, 97, 114–15
Smoking, 98–99, 108, 109, 173, 183, 186
Snoring, 115
Social connections and support, 191–93
Soluble fiber, 179–80
Sorghum, 173
Soy products, 161, 163, 175
Sperm count, low, 40
Sports massage, 199
Steroids, 46, 99, 101, 102, 151
Stillbirth, 129
Stress, 50, 120, 200
Stretching, 188–90
Strokes, 107, 108, 109, 110, 115, 184
Subacute viral thyroiditis. *See* De Quervain's (subacute viral) thyroiditis
Subclinical hypothyroidism, 1, 21, 26, 116, 118, 120, 127, 128
Subclinical thyrotoxicosis, 42
Sucralfate, 163
Sudden Infant Death Syndrome, 77
Sun exposure, 113

Support groups, online, 192
Surgery. *See also* Thyroidectomy
    for autonomous toxic nodules (ATNs), 72, 73
    for follicular thyroid cancer, 89
    for medullary thyroid cancer (MTC), 87
    for papillary thyroid cancer, 89, 90
    parathyroid gland damage by, 8–9, 93–94
    for toxic multinodular goiters, 74
Swedish massage, 199
Sweet potatoes, 173

T1, 157
T2, 157
T3. *See* Triiodothyronine (T3)
T4. *See* Thyroxine (T4)
Tachyarrhythmias, 107
Tachycardia, 111
Talk therapy, 106, 133, 195–97, 198
Tall cell papillary cancer, xiv, 85, 89
Tapazole. *See* Methimazole
Tears, artificial; in treating TED, 102
Technetium, 140
Testosterone, 40
Thiocyanates, 173
Three Mile Island, 137
ThyCa, 176
Thyrogen, 94, 95, 142, 143, 147
Thyroglobulin (Tg), 9, 59, 88
Thyroglobulin test (Tg test), 90, 94–95, 165, 166
Thyroid antibodies, 23, 24–25, 54, 122
Thyroid antibody tests, 54, 123
Thyroid bed, 148
Thyroid cancer, 1, 9, 12, 19, 52, 63, 64, 66, 68, 73, 74–75, 81–96, 117, 123–24, 140, 141–43, 153, 158, 160, 162, 191, 198
    anaplastic, 75, 87
    of author, xiii–xiv
    causes of, 81–83
    in children, 67, 81, 82
    deaths from, 81
    differentiated vs. undifferentiated, 88
    follicular (*see* Follicular thyroid cancer)
    follow-up scans and tests, 94–95
    Hurthle cell (oncocytic), 75, 86
    medullary (*see* Medullary thyroid cancer [MTC])
    papillary (*see* Papillary thyroid cancer)
    pregnancy and, 121, 130

radioactive iodine-induced (myth), 151
radioactive iodine therapy for, 86, 89,
    90, 92, 94–95, 138, 139, 143,
    146–50, 165–66, 170
rarity of, 81
screening for, 77–79
signs of, 83–84
staging and spreading, 87–88
treatment of, 89–90
treatment of recurrence, 96
types of, 85–87
unresponsive aggressive, 87
Thyroid disorders, 1, 9–12
after sixty, 118–20
women and, 36
Thyroid dysgenesis, 134
Thyroid dyshormonogenesis, 135
Thyroid eye disease (TED), 11, 46, 51,
    97–102
antithyroid medication and, 48
diabetes and, 44
diagnosis of, 101
Hashimoto's thyroiditis and, 24, 97
hot and cold phases of, 100
other names for, 37, 43, 97–98
radioactive iodine-induced (myth), 151
smoking and, 98–99
stages of, 101
symptoms of, 99–101
thyrotoxicosis and, 37, 98
treatment of, 101–2
Thyroid Federation International (TFI),
    22
Thyroid gland, 2–3
amount of iodine uptake by, 169
congenital absence of, 21, 135
ectopic, 134–35
enlarged, 16, 36–37 (*see also* Goiters)
hypoplastic, 135
iodine excess and, 172
weight of, 139
Thyroid hormone, 3, 59, 139, 169,
    170. *See also* Thyroxine (T4);
    Triiodothyronine (T3)
Thyroid hormone replacement, 12, 27,
    153–68
after sixty, 118–19
a brief history of, 154
de Quervain's thyroiditis and, 59
excessive dosage of, 10, 33, 51, 52,
    118–19
fiber supplements and, 179
following cancer therapy, 89, 90, 93

following Graves' disease therapy, 49
Hashimoto's thyroiditis and, 25–26
massage and, 199
misuse of, 52–53
morning sickness and, 124–25
natural, 119
postpartum, 132
pregnancy and, 128
silent thyroiditis and, 60
twenty-first-century, 157–64
Thyroid hormone resistance, 27, 29–30
Thyroid lobes. *See* Lobes, thyroid
Thyroid nodules. *See* Nodules, thyroid
Thyroid peroxidase (TPO), 25, 60, 61
Thyroid self-exam (TSE), 64–65, 78
Thyroid stare, 37
Thyroid storm, 42, 46
Thyroid surgery. *See* Surgery
Thyroidectomy
author's, xiv
for Graves' disease, 45, 48, 49
for Hashimoto's thyroiditis, 25–26
for malignant nodules, 75
near-total, 90, 91
partial, 49, 89, 90, 91
during pregnancy, 129
prophylactic, 83, 87
risks of, 91–94
for thyroid cancer, 90–94, 117, 153
total, xiv, 89, 90–91, 92, 94, 153
Thyroiditis, 53, 57–62, 139, 153
acute suppurative, 10, 61–62
amiodarone and, 164
de Quervain's (subacute viral), 10,
    57–59, 60
following thyroidectomy, 92
Hashimoto's (*see* Hashimoto's
    thyroiditis)
lymphocytic, 59
postpartum, 10, 60–61, 122, 127,
    131–33
prevalence of, 57
Riedel's, 62
silent, 10, 59–60, 131, 132
Thyroid-stimulating hormone (TSH), 3,
    16. *See also* Thyrogen; TSH test
autonomous toxic nodules (ATNs) and,
    51, 52, 63, 72, 73
Graves' disease and, 47, 48
Hashimoto's thyroiditis and, 23, 25
iodine and, 7, 170
in newborns, 122, 135, 136
radioactive iodine scans and, 142, 143

radioactive iodine therapy and, 147
reverse T3 and, 5–6
role of pituitary gland and, 6–7
subclinical hypothyroidism and, 26
suppression therapy, 52, 89, 90, 95–96,
    153, 158
thyroglobulin testing and, 95
thyroid cancer and, 88
thyrotoxicosis and, 54–55
Thyroid-stimulating immunoglobulin/
    antibody (TSI/TSA), 43, 45, 48, 101,
    126
Thyrotoxicity, 10, 183, 198
Thyrotoxicosis, 11, 20, 51–55, 72, 73,
    154, 184, 191
    after sixty, 118–19, 120
    amiodarone and, 164
    anxiety and, 102–3, 105–6
    burnout and, 116
    causes other than hyperthyroidism,
        51–53
    common causes of, 10
    diagnosing, 53–54
    fatigue and, 112, 113–14
    fetal, 126
    gestational, 124, 128
    heart disease and, 106, 108, 110–12
    hyperthyroidism distinguished from, 33
    menopause and, 116
    nonautoimmune, 98
    osteoporosis and, 116
    postpartum, 131
    radioactive iodine uptake test for, 139
    signs of, 33–43
    subclinical, 42
    thyroiditis and, 57, 58
    treatment for non-Graves' related,
        54–55
    yoga and, 190
Thyrotropin-releasing hormone (TRH), 7
Thyroxine (T4), 4, 38, 153, 154–68
    brand names vs. generics, 158–59
    combined with T3, 119, 155, 157,
        167–68
    conversion to T3 (*see* Conversion of T4
        to T3)
    dosage, 159–60
    drugs/supplements interfering with,
        162–64
    free (*see* Free T4 levels; Free T4 test;
        Free T3 test)
    Graves' disease and, 48
    half-life of, 165–66

how to take, 161–62
    in newborns, 134, 135
    pregnancy and, 125
    properties and effects of, 3
    storage and heat sensitivity, 160–61
    synthetic vs. natural, 154–57
    thyrotoxicosis and, 55
Thyroxine-binding globulin (TBG), 125,
    135
Tooth decay, 148
Toxic adenomas. *See* Autonomous toxic
    nodules (ATNs)
Toxic multinodular goiters, 51, 52, 63,
    73–74, 138
Tracheostomy, 92
Tremors, 41
Triglycerides, 181, 182, 188
Triiodothyronine (T3), 153, 154
    in bioidentical hormones, 117
    combined with T4, 119, 155, 157,
        167–68
    conversion from T4 (*see* Conversion of
        T4 to T3)
    facts about, 4
    free (test), 44, 53
    Graves' disease and, 48
    half-life of, 165–66, 167
    properties and effects of, 3
    reverse, 5–6
    for severe hypothyroidism, 166–67
    supplementation, necessary, 142,
        164–68 (*see also* Cytomel)
    supplementation, unnecessary, 4, 10,
        31
    thyrotoxicosis and, 20, 55
Trophoblastic neoplasia, gestational, 128
TSH. *See* Thyroid-stimulating hormone
    (TSH)
TSH test, 10
    after sixty, 118
    dosage of T4 and, 160
    false negative myth, 4
    generic vs. brand T4 and, 158
    Graves' disease diagnosed with, 44
    hyperthyroidism diagnosed with, 53
    hypothyroidism diagnosed with,
        19–21
    misunderstanding of, 20–21
    for nodules, 66
    postpartum depression and, 133
    pregnancy and, 123, 124, 125, 127–28
    thyrotoxicosis diagnosed with, 53
    truth about, 22

TSI/TSA. *See* Thyroid-stimulating immunoglobulin/antibody (TSI/TSA)
Tuina massage, 199
Turnips, 173
Twenty-four-hour radioactive iodine uptake, 140

Ukraine (radioactive fallout in), 82
Ultrasound, 66–68, 78, 101, 141
UNICEF, 171
Unipolar depression, 103–5
University of Kentucky, xv
University of Texas M.D. Anderson Cancer Center, 152
Unrestricted medical grants, 209

Vitamins, 162, 174, 175, 183
   A, 19, 183
   D, 8, 93, 94, 183
   E, 183
   prenatal, 124, 125
Vitiligo, 44
Vocal cord nerve damage, 92–93
Voice changes, 19
Volpé, Robert, xv
Volunteerism, 193

Water intake with fiber, 179, 180
Weight gain, 187. *See also* Obesity
   hypothyroidism and, 15–16
   with normal TSH levels, 31–32

Weight loss
   diet and, 181–83
   thyrotoxicosis and, 41, 184
Weight Watchers, 178
Whole body scans (WBS), 138, 141–43, 148, 165
Wilson, Denis E., 31
Wilson's thyroid syndrome, xviii, 30, 31
Women. *See also* Menopause; Menstrual cycle; Perimenopause; Pregnancy; Premenstrual syndrome (PMS)
   de Quervain's thyroiditis in, 58
   depression in, 104
   Graves' disease in, 43
   Hashimoto's thyroiditis in, 23, 57
   hypothyroidism in, 13
   infertility and, 122
   insomnia in, 115
   panic attacks in, 54
   psychiatric misdiagnoses in, 36
   silent thyroiditis in, 60
   thyroid cancer in, 81, 85, 86
   thyrotoxicosis in, 41
World Health Organization, 134, 171

X-rays, 140

Yoga, 190

Zinc, 172

About the Author

M. SARA ROSENTHAL, Ph.D., is a pioneer in consumer health writing. She began her career as a journalist, and her interest in health issues arose from her experience with thyroid cancer in 1983. She first published *The Thyroid Sourcebook* in 1993, which was recommended by the *New York Times*. Over the years, Dr. Rosenthal has written more than thirty consumer health books, and she has been the publisher of many more through her own consumer health publishing company, Your Health Press (yourhealthpress.com). Her books are translated into several languages including Arabic, Chinese, Polish, Russian, Spanish, and Taiwanese.

In 1996 Dr. Rosenthal became interested in bioethics as a result of her patient advocacy work, and she pursued an academic career in bioethics. She completed her master's and doctorate in bioethics at the University of Toronto Joint Centre for Bioethics. She is currently a bioethicist at the University of Kentucky; as an academician, she publishes on endocrine ethics in the peer-reviewed literature.

Dr. Rosenthal is a member of the American Society for Bioethics and Humanities, The American Thyroid Association, and The Endocrine Society. She serves on the Advisory Panel of Ethics and Conflict of Interest as a member of the Endocrine Society as well as the Patient Education and Advocacy Committee of the American Thyroid Association.